MUSCULOSKELETAL MANIPULATION

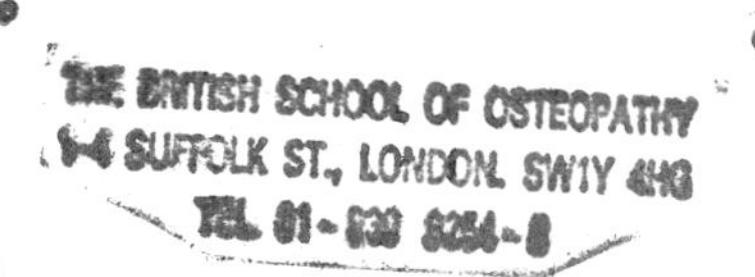

MUSCULOSKELETAL MANIPULATION

Evaluation of the Scientific Evidence

By

JEROME S. TOBIS, M.D.

Professor and former Chairman
Department of Physical Medicine and Rehabilitation
and
Director, Program in Geriatric Medicine
California College of Medicine
University of California, Irvine
Irvine, California

and

FRED HOEHLER, Ph.D.

Director
Technical Information Services
Newport Pharmaceuticals International, Incorporated
Newport Beach, California
and
Assistant Clinical Professor
Department of Physical Medicine and Rehabilitation
California College of Medicine
University of California, Irvine
Irvine, California

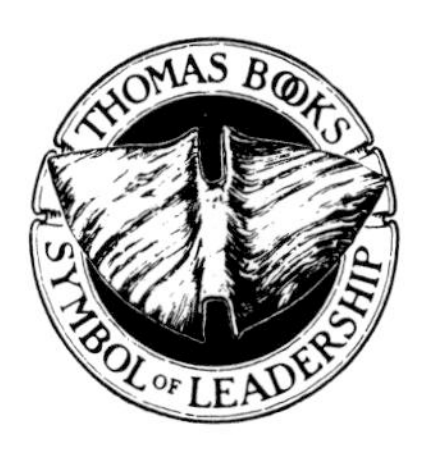

CHARLES C THOMAS • PUBLISHER
Springfield • Illinois • U.S.A.

Published and Distributed Throughout the World by

CHARLES C THOMAS • PUBLISHER
2600 South First Street
Springfield, Illinois 62717

ISBN 0-398-05198-4

Library of Congress Catalog Card Number: 85-20864

With THOMAS BOOKS *careful attention is given to all details of manufacturing and design. It is the Publisher's desire to present books that are satisfactory as to their physical qualities and artistic possibilities and appropriate for their particular use.* THOMAS BOOKS *will be true to those laws of quality that assure a good name and good will.*

Printed in the United States of America
Q-R-3

Library of Congress Cataloging in Publication Data

Tobis, Jerome S.
Musculoskeletal manipulation.

Bibliography: p.
Includes index.
1. Manipulation (Therapeutics) I. Hoehler, Fred.
II. Title.
RM724.T63 1986 615.8'2 85-20864
ISBN 0-398-05198-4

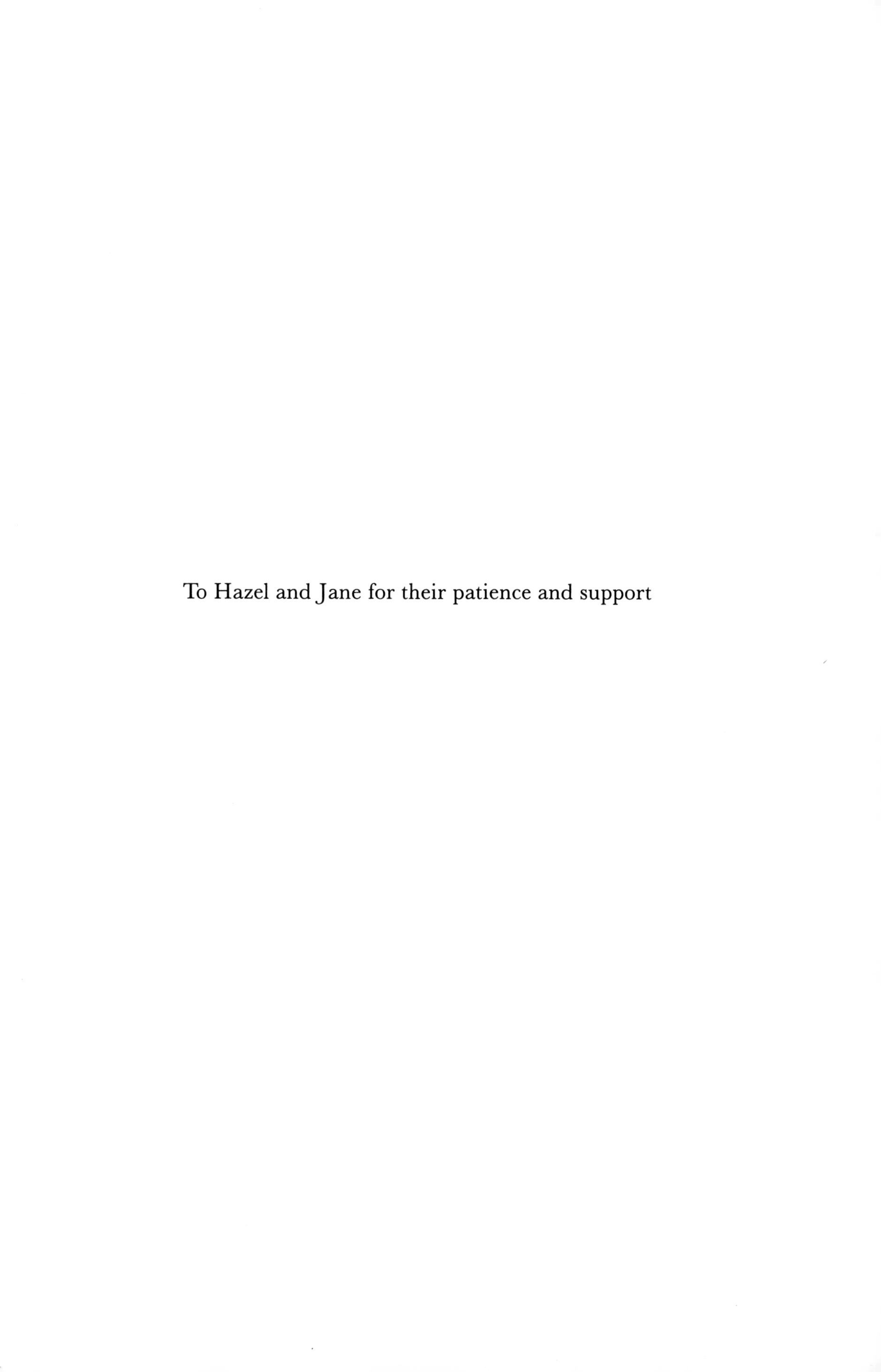

To Hazel and Jane for their patience and support

PREFACE

THIS MONOGRAPH has had a long history in its conception and ultimate birth. The project is the result of a research and clinical program that began to develop in 1970 at the California College of Medicine of the University of California. One of the authors (JST) joined the faculty as Chairman of the Department of Physical Medicine and Rehabilitation at that time, attracted by the challenge of an allopathic medical school interested in studying the efficacy of Musculoskeletal Manipulation as a therapeutic modality for back pain. Historically the school had been an osteopathic institution prior to its amalgamation with the University of California educational system and thus was unique among public medical schools at that time.

There were many former osteopaths who were alumni of the College who were enthusiastic to undertake such a research program. The individual whose leadership and perseverence facilitated the establishment of the research is Forest Grunigen, M.D. His support facilitated the long-term funding of the project by the Forty-first Medical Trust. In this regard, the authors wish to express appreciation to the former dean of the school, Stanley van den Noort, M.D., whose enthusiasm and interest in the project enabled it to come to fruition. Dr. Alfred Buerger is another former colleague who deserves special recognition in the development of the program. He was associated with us for several years in the study.

The second author (FH) joined the project after the first few years of its development and has been associated with it throughout its history.

This study was reported in scientific literature beginning in 1977 (Buerger and Tobis, 1977). Subsequently a series of papers have been published recording our data and experience.

Incidentally, we believe our study was the first controlled clinical trial of manipulation to be reported in the United States.

This monograph thus, in part, represents a summing up of our experience and interpretation of the data we had obtained from the study. However, it is intended to provide more than that. We have attempted to review and analyze all of the published reports that have appeared in refereed journals concerning trials evaluating spinal manipulation. Further we have given a brief background concerning the history of manipulation. It has been employed for centuries with the use of many different techniques and it is likely to continue to be part of the armamentarium for treatment of low back pain for a long time to come.

Other subjects that are included in this volume deal with the etiological factors of back pain, specific techniques that are currently employed by prominent practitioners of manipulation as well as indications for manipulation and theories concerning its effectiveness.

We hope that this report will be a stimulus for other investigators to pursue new studies that may answer the many important questions concerning this fascinating subject.

Research performed at the University of California Irvine Medical Center was supported by a grant from 41st Medical Trust, Los Angeles.

This project was supervised by a coordinating committee that consisted of J. E. Berk, M.D., A. A. Buerger, Ph.D., T. Crocker, M.D., G. Gordon, M.D., F. Grunigen, M.D., H. Guirgis, Ph.D., S. Haldeman, Ph.D., M.D., W. Hopps, M.D., J. Kusske, M.D., A. Starr, M.D., J. Swett, M.D., R. F. Thompson, Ph.D., J. Tobis, M.D., and S. van den Noort, M.D., The back clinic was staffed by W. Dooley, M.D., E. Evans, M.D., A. Fulmor, M.D., C. Garrett, M.D., F. Grunigen, M.D., E. Hackler, R.N., W. Hopps, M.D., E. Houghtaling, M.D., C. Johnson, M.D., E. Privett, R.N., P.H.N. and Peter Van Etten, M.D.

We want to thank
Phyllis Wood and Susan Vega
for their valuable assistance
in the transcription of the text

CONTENTS

MUSCULOSKELETAL MANIPULATION

CHAPTER I

AN HISTORICAL PERSPECTIVE OF MANIPULATION

IN 1975, the National Institute of Neurological Diseases and Stroke of the prestigious National Institutes of Health held a "Workshop on the Research Status of Spinal Manipulative Therapy." The establishment of such a conference with the subsequent publication of its proceedings (Goldstein, 1975a) signifies the level of scientific inquiry which this therapeutic modality of manipulation has attained.

The history of manipulative therapy is filled with charges and countercharges of charlatanry and deceit, of claims and counterclaims of efficacy for a multitude of medical conditions. Such heated arguments are of relatively recent vintage. However, through the ages, both orthodox physicians and folk practitioners in Europe and the Middle East wrote about the value of manipulation for the treatment of acute back pain (Goldstein, 1975). According to Goldstein:

> "It seems probable that the genesis of the modern theory and practice of manipulative therapy as used by chiropractors, osteopathic physicians and medical physicians arose from concepts generally acceptable to many eminent 19th century medical practitioners and scientists since it was during this period that the role of the spinal cord in health and disease was being vigorously explored and discussed."

Lomax (1977) describes spinal manipulation as an ancient art, sanctioned by Hippocrates and practiced widely until the 18th century. Cyriax (1982) claims that Hippocrates in the fifth century B.C. and Galen in the third century A.D. both practiced this art. Others, including Avicenna in the tenth century and Paré in the sixteenth century taught manipulative techniques.

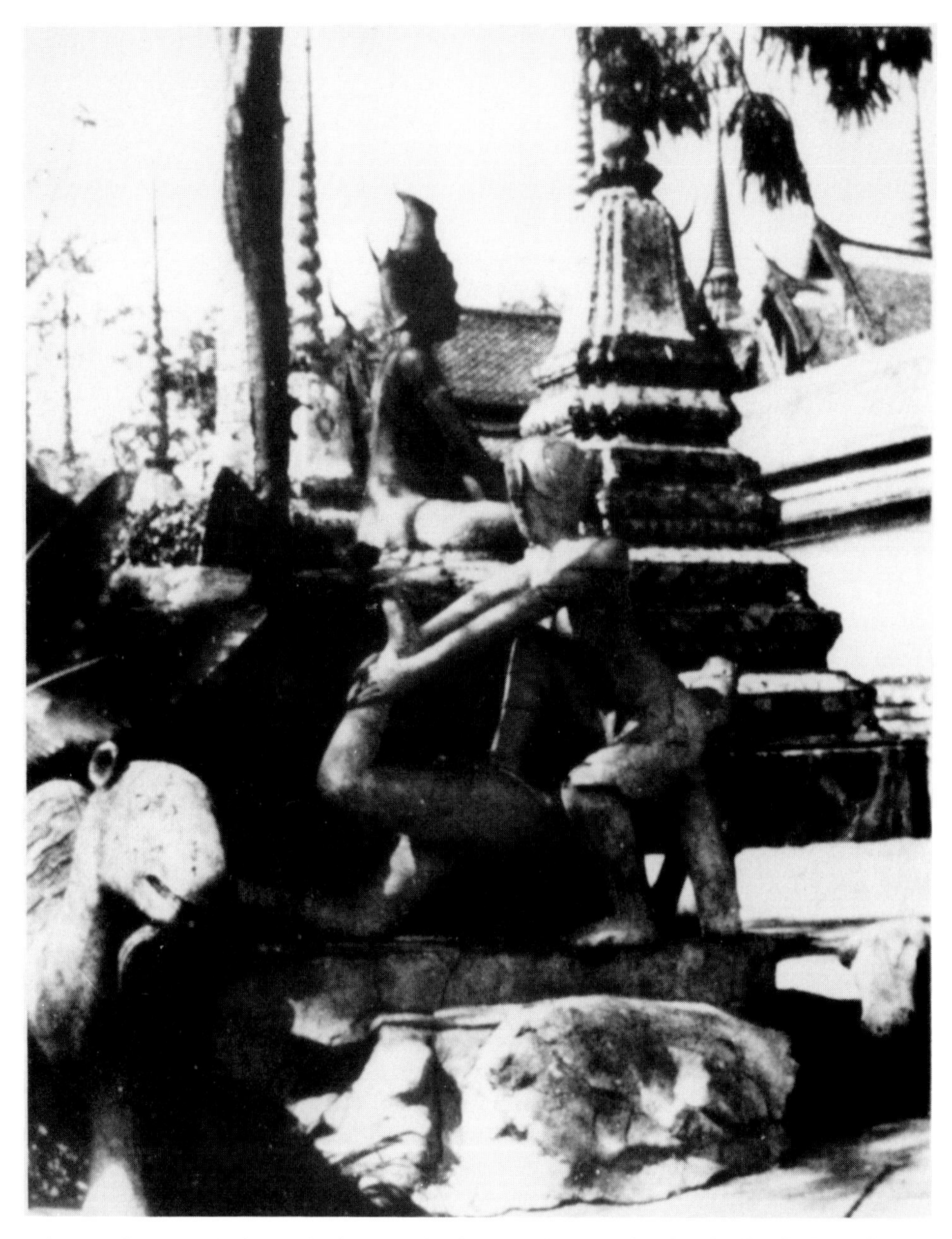

Figure I-1. An early form of spinal manipulation. Photograph taken by Dr. K.I. Mah at an ancient Buddhist Temple at Bangkok, Siam and regarded as 2000 years old (from Schiotz and Cyriax, 1975).

According to Schiotz and Cyriax (1975) manipulation has been part of folk medicine of many nations for innumerable generations (see Figure I-1). In Central Europe, gypsies have possessed the ability to cure acute lumbago by manipulation. Some people in Tibet, as well as in Japan, have developed techniques of manipulation for treating musculoskeletal complaints of the back. The "stamping" cure consisted of a woman standing "with both feet on the invalid's back and trampling up and down. Or she might walk across—or up and down—his back."

Another form of musculoskeletal manipulation was practised since time immemorial by bonesetters in Germany, France, Scandinavia and Great Britain. Often their methods were transmitted as family secrets from one generation to the next.

During the 18th century, tuberculosis of the spine was identified as a contraindication to its use. "Since then," Lomax states, "spinal manipulation has had a checkered career among orthopedists, retained by a few as a helpful technique when used with circumspection, but rejected by a majority as nonspecific, unscientific and tainted with quackery."

From Hippocrates through Galen, Celsus, Oribasius, Albucasis and Paré, the employment of manipulation was condoned so long as certain admonitions were abided. In the latter portion of the 18th century, Potts' descriptions of spinal caries were published, influencing many physicians to believe that all curvatures of the spine were due to disease of the bones and therefore condemning manipulation as dangerous. This group, as a consequence, viewed manipulation as a form of malpractice and the bonesetters' activities were severely criticized.

There were, of course, exceptions to the large group of disclaimers. Such was Edward Harrison who maintained a successful practice in London from 1817 until his death in 1838. Others included Andrew Dods in 1821 and William John Little in 1868.

A diagnosis of "spinal irritation" began to assume a prominent role in the etiology of innumerable complaints sometime after 1828 when it was first described by Thomas Brown of Glasgow. Subsequently, in the 19th century there were few complaints that could not be explained as related to the spinal column. Is it possible that this theory may have influenced Andrew Taylor Still, the founder of osteopathy?

According to Bordley and Harvey (1976) the cult of osteopathy began to develop in Andrew Still's mind during the 1860s. His observations of the inadequacy of medicine of that era included the inability to cure infections and alter diseases and also criticized the employment of drugs that were ineffective and dangerous. In 1874, he announced the use of spinal manipulation as a new system of therapy.

In 1895, D. O. Palmer, a self-styled healer in Davenport, Iowa founded a new cult of chiropractic medicine which, too, was based on the tenet that the best treatment for any disease is spinal manipulation. In spite of many professional obstacles, the field has prospered and grown.

Today, manipulation is practised by thousands of osteopaths, chiropractors, physicians, and physical therapists throughout the world.

Currently, chiropractors are most prominent in the treatment of back and neck pain. Kane et al (1964) examined the records of the Utah State Workmen's Compensation fund for 1972 and found that chiropractors treated 28% of the 795 cases of back and neck injury. Comparisons of patients treated by chiropractors with a random sample of patients treated by physicians indicated that the chiropractic patients had a shorter duration of treatment (6.5 vs 9.3 weeks) but a greater number of visits to the therapist (12.8 vs 7.3). Eighty percent of them reported complete functional improvement as compared to 70 percent of the patients treated by physicians. Chiropractic patients also reported more satisfaction in the ability of the practitioner to make the patient feel welcome (100% vs 94%) and to explain the problem and treatment (95% vs 84%). Dvorak (1983) has recently surveyed the field of manual medicine in the United States and has found that there are approximately 23,000 chiropractors and 19,000 osteopaths currently practicing manipulative therapy. A relatively small number of physicians (approximately 250) are members of the North American Academy of Manipulative Medicine. Obviously, manipulative therapy is a popular and frequently employed therapeutic modality. The purpose of this book will be to examine and evaluate the scientific evidence regarding this form of treatment.

CHAPTER II

THEORIES OF THE CAUSE OF FUNCTIONAL BACK PAIN

STRICTLY SPEAKING, back pain is not a specific disease entity. Rather,it is a symptom and, as such, may be the result of a wide variety of pathological conditions.

The multiplicity of possible causes of back pain is displayed in Table II-1 and we do not wish to imply that even this is complete. However, in terms of frequency, mechanical and psychological factors alone, or in a combination, contribute to the vast majority of complaints described by patients.

As shown in Figure II-1, the nature of the uncomplicated low back pain has been estimated to clear up in 90% of all cases within three weeks.

It sometimes seems as though there are as many theories of the etiology of nonspecific low back pain as there are practitioners who treat this disorder. Virtually every structure impinging on the spinal column has been implicated (see Figure II-2).

In this chapter, we shall attempt to describe some of the major theories. We should, however, reiterate the rather commonplace observation that it is quite unlikely that any of these theories will explain all cases of nonspecific back pain. It simply may not be reasonable to assume that back pain results from a single mechanism (Haldeman, 1977a; 1977b; Flor and Turk, 1984).

The General Theories—Osteopathy and Chiropractic

Osteopathic and chiropractic theories of back pain are most interesting to one concerned with either the history of medical science or contemporary medical politics. Osteopathy developed from the ideas of

Table II-1

ETIOLOGIC FACTORS IN LOW BACK PAIN

I. Congenital disorders
   A. Facet tropism (asymmetry)
   B. Transitional vertebra
      1. Sacralization of lumbar vertebra
II. Tumors
   A. Benign
      1. Tumors involving nerve roots or meninges (e.g., neurinoma, hemangioma, meningioma)
      2. Tumors involving vertebrae (e.g., osteoid osteoma, Paget's disease, osteoblastoma)
   B. Malignant
      1. Primary bone tumors (e.g., multiple myeloma)
      2. Primary neural tumors
      3. Secondary tumors (e.g., metastases from breast, prostate, kidney, lung, thyroid)
III. Trauma
   A. Lumbar strain
      1. Acute
      2. Chronic
   B. Compression fracture
      1. Fracture of vertebral body
      2. Fracture of transverse process
   C. Subluxated facet joint (facet syndrome)
   D. Spondylolysis and spondylolisthesis
IV. Toxicity
   A. Heavy metal poisoning (e.g., radium)
V. Metabolic disorders (e.g., osteoporosis)
VI. Inflammatory diseases (e.g., rheumatoid arthritis, ankylosing spondylitis)
VII. Degenerative disorders (e.g., spondylosis, osteoarthritis, herniated disc, herniated nucleus pulposus, spinal stenosis — nerve root entrapment syndrome)
VIII. Infections
   A. Acute (e.g., pyogenic disc space infections)
   B. Chronic (e.g., tuberculosis, chronic osteomyelitis, fungal infection)
IX. Circulatory disorders (e.g., abdominal aortic aneurysm)
X. Mechanical causes
   A. Intrinsic (e.g., poor muscle tone, chronic postural strain, myofascial pain, unstable vertebrae)
   B. Extrinsic (e.g., uterine fibroids, pelvic tumors or infections, hip diseases, prostate disease, sacroiliac joint infections and sprains, untreated lumbar scoliosis)
XI. Psychoneurotic problems (e.g., hysteria, malingering, compensatory low back pain — "green poultice" syndrome)

From Keim and Kirkaldy-Willis (1980)

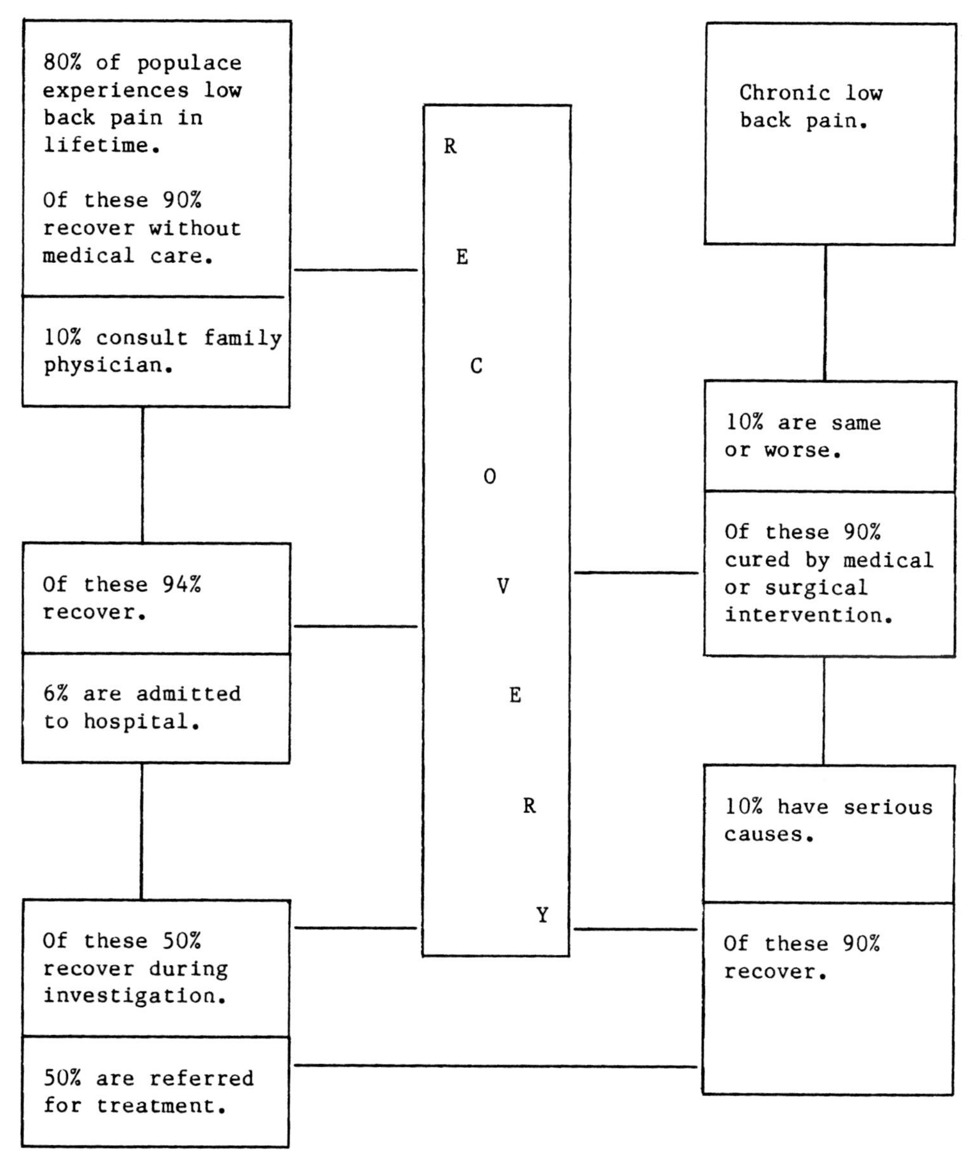

Figure II-1. Estimated outcomes of back pain in an English population (modified from Dixon, 1976).

Andrew Taylor Still (1910) in the 1860s, who maintained that all disease results from displacements of the vertebrae. These displacements tend to impair circulation or nervous transmission and, thus, may produce disease in any organ of the body. Currently, osteopaths palpate the spinal column searching for muscle spasm or areas of restricted or painful range of motion. This is referred to as the "osteopathic lesion" and is believed to be the major cause of nonspecific back pain (Denslow, 1975).

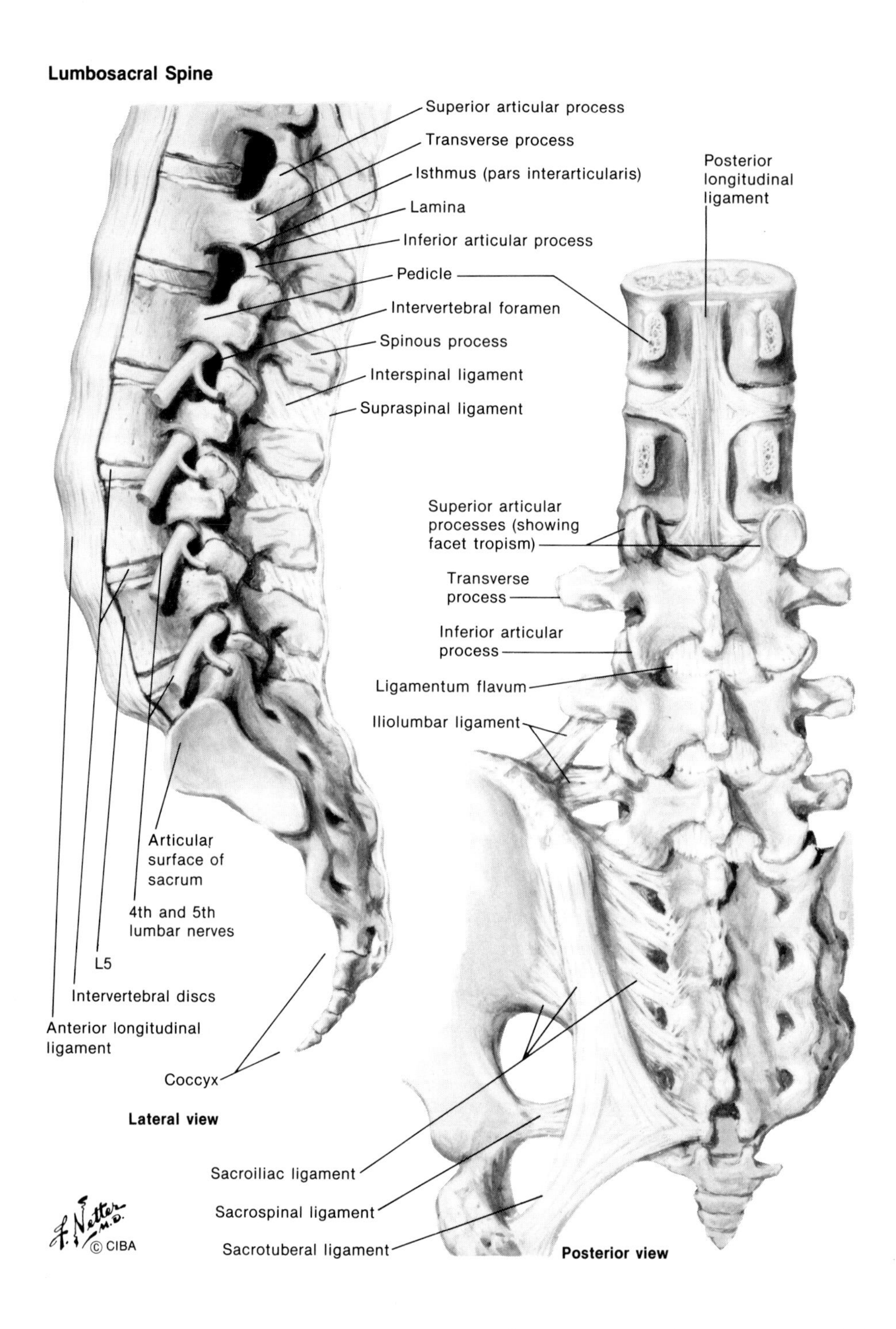

Figure II-2. Anatomy of the lumbar sacral spine. ©Copyright 1980 CIBA Pharmaceutical Company, Division of CIBAGEIGY Corporation. Reprinted with permission from CLINICAL SYMPOSIA, illustrated by Frank H. Netter, M.D. All rights reserved.

Hoag (1969) states that "An osteopathic lesion is a musculoskeletal disorder which, by its presence, either instigates, augments or maintains an alteration in function of some tissue of the body. The classic type of osteopathic lesion is represented by an abnormality in spinal mobility—usually a partial or complete restriction of motion, but at least an altered pattern of motion between vertebral segments."

In most states of this country, osteopaths are now permitted to prescribe drugs and perform surgery (Wardwell, 1972) and, therefore, they have largely abandoned the notion that most or all disease is attributable to spinal subluxations and curable by spinal manipulation.

Chiropractic manipulative techniques and theories were developed somewhat later than osteopathy and are, in many respects, quite similar (Palmer, 1934). Like the early osteopaths, chiropractors believe that small vertebral displacements can produce nonspecific back pain as well as many other symptoms and that pain can be alleviated by adjustment of those displaced vertebrae. Unlike the osteopaths, chiropractors have remained well outside orthodox medicine (Firman & Goldstein, 1975) and still prescribe spinal manipulation for the treatment of a wide variety of disorders.

The Intervertebral Disc

Goldthwait (1911) was perhaps the first to suggest that back pain with sciatica was caused by the pressure exerted by a herniated intervertebral disc on the nerve roots that join to form the sciatic nerve. Later studies by Mixter and Barr (1934) convincingly demonstrated the existence of a syndrome characterized by nerve root entrapment produced by a herniated disc.

Because the herniated nucleus pulposus is a known cause of back pain, it was to be expected that many cases of nonspecific back pain would be attributed to some lesion of the disc. Some type of disc pathology appears to be a virtually universal phenomenon of aging. In several large series, the proportion of the population with some variety of radiographically detectable disc degeneration is quite high and is a direct function of age rising to 60% in the 60 years and over age group (Horal, 1969; Hult, 1954) (see Figure II-3).

These are not herniated discs, and although there is some correlation between degenerative disc lesions and back pain, it is not particularly high. Many people with radiographically demonstrated disc degeneration have no back pain and many people with back pain have no disc

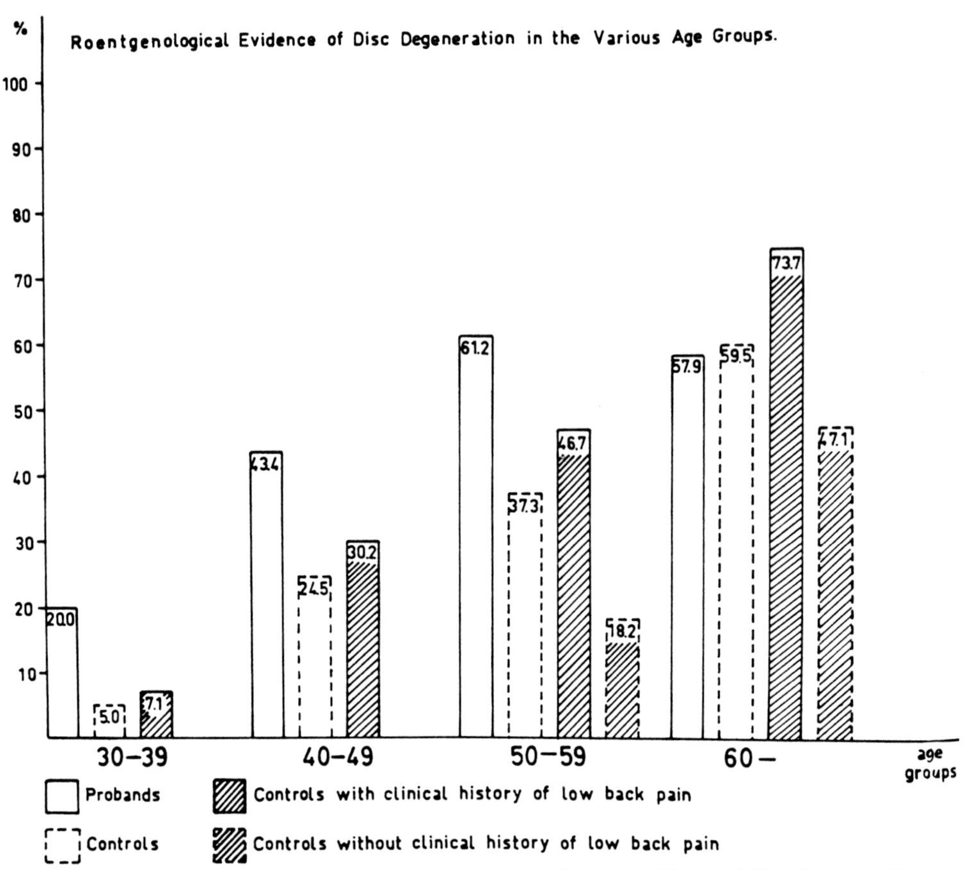

Figure II-3. Percentage of individuals with roentgenological evidence of disc degeneration as a function of age and clinical history of back pain (from Hult, 1957).

degeneration. Therefore, it seems unlikely that this type of lesion is a direct cause of all back pain. It is more likely that the factors which produce disc degeneration also tend to produce back pain in some individuals. However, because it was known that a herniated disc can produce back pain and, because most patients above a certain age will have demonstrable lesions of the disc, many cases of back pain have been misdiagnosed as being of discogenic origin, and a large amount of unnecessary surgery has been performed. In these cases, surgery is not only useless, it is likely to exacerbate the back pain and can, in fact, cause a sciatic syndrome through the development of nerve root adhesions (Fahrni, 1966). Perhaps for this reason, several studies have failed to demonstrate that surgery has any significant long-term beneficial effect except on back pain of specific etiologies (Armstrong, 1982; Spongfort, 1972; Frymoyer et al, 1978). A recent randomized prospective study of surgical vs conservative treatment of patients with herniated lumbar discs verified by radiculopathy showed that, even in this population, statistically significant beneficial effects of surgery were only observed at the one-year follow-up and were not apparent at four and ten years (Weber, 1983).

In a similar fashion, this type of misdiagnosis may have impeded the use of chemonucleolysis in the treatment of herniated nucleus pulposus. Chemonucleolysis involves the injection of a proteolytic enzyme, such as chymopapain, into the intervertebral space in an attempt to dissolve the offending fragments of disc. Early studies indicated the utility of this treatment (Ford, 1969; McNab et al, 1971) but a multicenter double-blind clinical trial showed no difference between interdiscal injections of chymopapain vs. placebo (Schwetschenau et al, 1976). However, more recent clinical trials have shown that, if the patient population is strictly limited to those with a proven herniated disc, a significant beneficial effect of chemonucleolysis is found (Javid et al, 1983). It appears that, like surgery, chemonucleolysis is only useful in the treatment of a truly prolapsed disc and may not be beneficial in the great majority of cases of nonspecific back pain.

Despite the failure of surgery or chemonucleolysis to alleviate many cases of back pain, there is still some support for the hypothesis that the source of most back pain is attributable to lesions of the intervertebral disc. Cyriax (1971, 1982) has long contended that back pain often results from a displaced fragment of intervertebral disc that may cause local pain by preventing the free movement of joints or may, through nerve root compression, cause pain elsewhere in the body. A disc that is not herniated or does not impinge on other surrounding structures might also be a source of pain. Smyth and Wright (1958) have reported that mechanical irritation (produced by nylon threads fastened during previous surgery) to the annulus fibrosus or the dorsal longitudinal ligament was capable of eliciting "sciatic" pain. Irritation of the lumbosacral fascia, the interspinous ligaments, the intervertebral joints or the ligamentum flavum had no such effect. It has also been reported that the interdiscal injection of hypertonic saline (Holt, 1968; Hirsh, 1966; 1978) or other stimulation of the disc (Cloward, 1960; Falconer et al 1978) can elicit pain similar to that experienced in attacks of back pain. Thus, it appears possible that the disc may be the source of pain in at least some cases of nonspecific back pain.

The Articulations

Both the facet joints and the ligaments of the spinal column (see Figure II-2) have been implicated in the etiology of the nonspecific back pain. Hypotheses involving the facet joints have been particularly popular as explanations of back pain treatable by spinal manipulation because manipulation typically involves gapping of those joints. This produces the characteristic popping sound that many manipulators believe to be a sign that the manuever has been properly executed. Several possible lesions of the facet joints may result in back pain. These are: (1) impacted synovial membrane (2) facet joint impaction (Cailliet, 1968) (3) entrapment of a meniscoid body (Lewit, 1978) (4) entrapment of a loose body and (5) sprain of the capsular ligament. All but the last of these would be expected to respond rapidly to manipulation.

The interspinous ligaments were first implicated in back pain by Kellgren (1939) who injected hypertonic saline into the midline of the back and produced pain of a segmental distribution similar to sciatica. Steindler (1948) noted that this pain could be eliminated by local anesthesia of the area of the lesion. However, it has been noted that the saline injection technique produces too diffuse an area of irritation to clearly implicate one particular structure (Sinclair et al, 1948). A further problem with hypotheses involving the facet joints as well as the ligaments is that the putative lesion is not clearly defined. Such lesions as are observed in the facets (Lewit, 1978) and the ligaments (Nachemson and Evans, 1968) appear to be secondary to disc degeneration.

The Muscles and Fascia

Hypotheses of the myofascial genesis of back pain go back at least as far as Gowers (1904). These theories usually involve the mechanism of the pain cycle in which an initial stimulus produces pain and that pain produces a reflex muscle spasm which maintains the pain indefinitely. Manipulation presumably interrupts this cycle of pain. Theories differ in the nature of the proposed initiating stimulus which may be a myofascial trigger point (Travell and Rinzler, 1952), fear of injury (Sarno, 1981) or minor intervertebral derangements (Maigne, 1972). The mechanism for the indefinite maintenance of pain has been somewhat less clearly defined but contraction-induced ischemia, which prevents the removal of toxic pain and fatigue-inducing substances, has often been mentioned (Travell and Rinzler, 1952; Sarno, 1981). Pain-induced spasm might also produce a long-lasting change in the "gain" of the muscle spindles such that the stretch reflex is evoked by any tendency towards relaxation (Korr, 1974).

These theories are quite difficult to test directly. Electromyographic investigations of back pain patients have generally shown increased electrical activity of the paravertebral muscles (DeVries, 1968; Kravitz et al, 1981; Hoyt et al, 1981), but this does not clearly implicate a myofascial reflex cycle as the cause of back pain, because pain generated elsewhere in the spinal region would also be expected to maintain a reflex muscle spasm.

It is apparent that we know little about the etiology of functional back pain. However, we need not let this ignorance concerning the cause of back pain prevent us from undertaking research on the treatment of that pain by spinal manipulation. Indeed, it is possible that clinical studies of manipulation may teach us more about the basic causes of back pain than basic research will teach us about manipulation.

CHAPTER III

TECHNIQUES OF MANIPULATION

MANY DIFFERENT theories have been proposed to explain the rationale for manipulation based upon the particular school one espouses. With so many different approaches, one would presume that there are wide differences among the techniques of various manipulators.

In practice, however, it would appear that all methods are empirical and there is a wide overlap of maneuvers employed by all. Perhaps the greatest difference in technique resides in the intensity of the force applied. Thus they extend from the gentle to the very powerful thrust.

Beal (1982) employs the term "the barrier of resistance" to joint movement as the basis for classifying osteopathic techniques as direct, indirect, and combined procedures. Direct techniques use operator forces against the barrier. Indirect techniques, on the other hand, lead the manipulator's applied force away from the barrier.

According to Fisk (1977b) the principle involved in most techniques "is to position the patient in such a way that a short sharp thrust can be applied to the facet joints." This maneuver is generally described as a high velocity, short amplitude technique. "The joints must be as near to right angles to their surface as anatomically possible, and in full apposition to each other, neither flexed nor extended." Fisk states that the aim of most techniques is to localize a rotational force at the level of a lesion or symptom. "In the lumbar spine there may be a long and a short lever. The purpose of the long lever is to hold the vertebrae above the joint to be manipulated while a high-velocity short-amplitude thrust is applied to the joint through the short lever." Fisk describes some five different techniques for the lumbar region.

Maigne (1972) divides the techniques of manipulation into three types. In the first method, pressure is applied directly to the spine and is designated a direct method. In the indirect method, the maneuvers are performed indirectly "through the natural levers formed by hand, shoulders, pelvis and legs, the spine being moved through their intermediary." The third method, Maigne designates as semi-direct because the manipulator stabilizes the part directly.

In the direct technique, the force is applied through the pisiform bone and the heel of the hand. The force is abrupt. In the indirect and semi-indirect maneuvers, it is important that the preparatory stages consist of positioning the patient and taking up the "slack."

Cyriax is convinced that the primary cause of low back pain is due to disc lesions causing degenerative change and pain of spinal origin. Therefore, the objective of the technique he employs is to reduce a small intraarticular displacement of cartilage.

Cyriax (1971) has described five different types of manipulation. These he designates as osteopathy, chiropractic, bonesetting, oscillatory techniques and the methods evolved by himself. Cyriax proposes that osteopaths lock the facet joints before manipulating the involved spinal joint. He claims that, in general, osteopaths force a joint by distant leverage, whereas chiropractors apply their pressure directly to the bone itself. The latter tend to apply a strong thrust at one particular joint.

Bonesetters, according to Cyriax are largely unschooled manipulators and represent a craft in Britain that is centuries old and skills that have been handed down through generations. The technique consists of applying a maneuver near where the symptom is experienced.

Oscillatory techniques consist of anterior-posterior pressures and releases to the affected joint as the patient lies prone. Lateral oscillations can also be applied. The manipulator places both thumbs on the top of the involved spinous process and applies his oscillations at the rate of about two per second. Both elbows are flexed and extended synchronously so that a series of little thrusts is delivered to the bone.

In the technique devised by Cyriax, a series of spinal joints is moved to its extreme range, the normal joints move freely, the blocked joint cannot. "The unaffected joints are thus moved as far as they can go now. The final overpressure falls inevitably on the deranged joint. Moving the normal joints is carried out gradually over a wide range and continued until the resistance of the blocked joint makes itself felt. Then a final thrust of tiny amplitude is given acting on the displacement itself." Many of these maneuvers are carried out during traction.

Lumbar Manipulation

Kirkaldy-Willis (1983) has defined lumbar manipulation as "a passive manual maneuver during which the three joint complex is suddenly carried beyond the normal physiological range of movement without exceeding the boundaries of anatomical integrity." The stages of manipulation are shown in Figure III-l which shows the four "zones" of movement of a joint. At the end of the range of passive motion "elastic barriers" of resistance are felt. Forcing the joint beyond this barrier produces a sudden yielding and, often, a cracking noise. Forcing motion beyond the final barrier would produce traumatic injury.

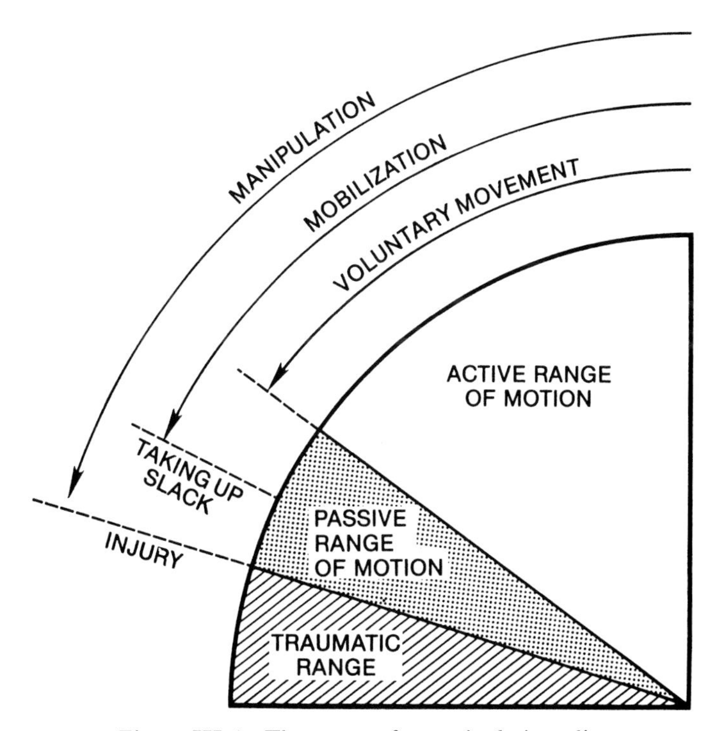

Figure III-1. The stages of a manipulative adjustment.

For lumbar vertebral manipulation, Maitland (1977) has described his method. "Maximum rotary stretch is applied by rocking the patient back and forth with the forearms, altering the position of the right forearm on the buttock if the lumbar spine position needs to be adjusted... The manipulation then consists of increasing the push through both forearms and sharply increasing the pressure against the adjacent spinous processes." This technique appears to coincide with the one described by Cyriax as "oscillatory."

In our research study on manipulation, the maneuver we employed coincides with an osteopathic technique and consisted of the patient lying on his or her side on a table facing the manipulator. The inferior leg

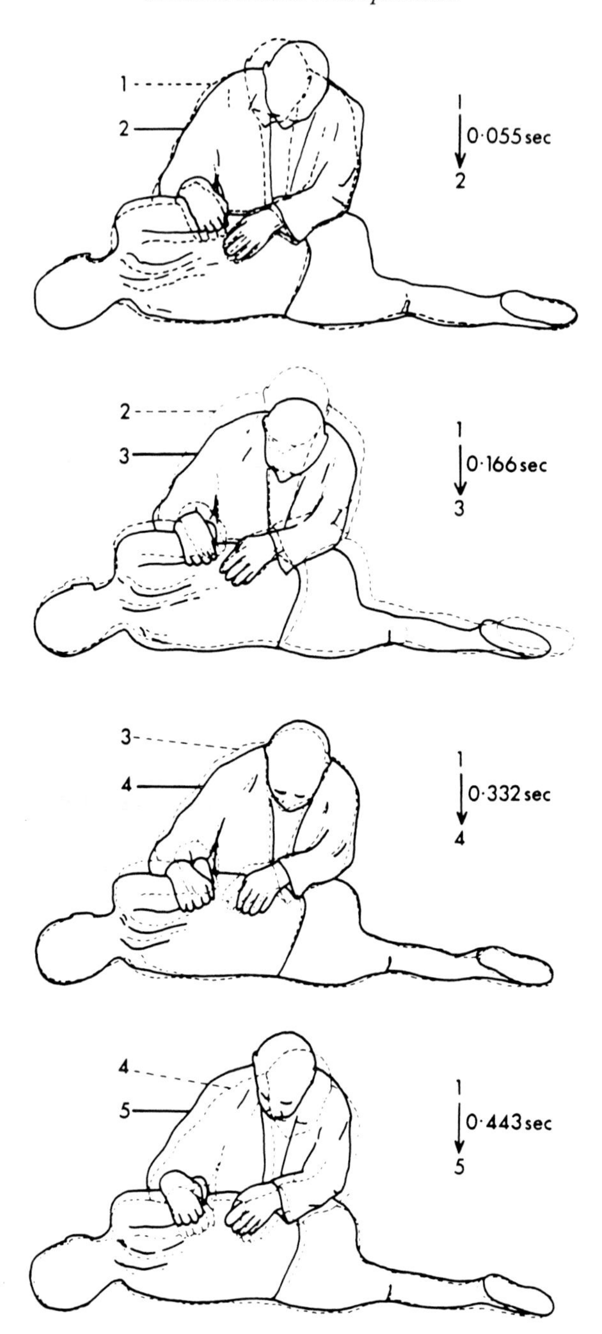

Figure III-2. Tracings from a filmed record of a rotational manipulation of the lumbosacral spine. Time intervals for each portion of the maneuver are shown.

is extended and the superior leg is flexed, tilting the superior aspect of the pelvis toward the manipulator. The superior shoulder is rotated away from the manipulator and the spine is "locked" in extension. A short, high velocity thrust is then applied to the pelvis (see Figure III-2).

The rationale for this maneuver is based on the assumption that there is "gapping" of the facet joints and stretching of the paravertebral muscles of the lumbosacral area.

Dorsal Manipulation

The first dorsal technique employed by Fisk (1977b) is accomplished by the patient lying supine with fingers locked behind the neck. The manipulator's farther arm is placed under the spine with the hand held clenched and as a fulcrum. With the other arm, pressure is applied to the flexed elbows with a downward thrust. This will result in distraction and gapping of the adjacent joints. This technique may be employed for joints between the third and eighth dorsal vertebrae.

The second dorsal vertebra technique is supplied by the pisiform bones of both hands providing short levers over the transverse processes of the vertebra below the joint. A sharp downward thrust is carried out, with the patient prone. Fisk claims this technique may be useful over the lower dorsal vertebrae.

Cervical Manipulation

With the patient in a supine position, transverse vertebral pressure may be applied to the atlas. The second metacarpophalangeal joint of the manipulator's hand may engage the lateral mass of the atlas. Lateral flexion of the patient's head may be carried out passively simultaneously (Grieve, 1979).

For movement of the axis, the patient is placed in a prone position and transverse vertebral pressure is directed toward the side of the pain.

Mobilization techniques may be applied to the lower cervical and upper thoracic segments which combine side flexion rotation and traction. Transverse pressures may be applied to adjacent spinous processes for the lower cervical and upper thoracic spinous processes.

One technique has been considered to be effective for manipulation of all the cervical spines except for the first. The patient is supine. The manipulator places one hand under the neck of the patient and the other hand under the chin. Rotation and side bend of the head is carried out. The slack is taken up at which point a short thrust is applied.

This summary of different manipulative techniques is not presented with the expectation that a reader will, as a result of the perusal of this chapter, be able to undertake any one procedure. To be an effective manipulator, one should observe numerous demonstrations of the procedures as performed by an experienced and informed instructor.

Many theories have been propounded to explain the rationale for the maneuvers that have been described. None, in our opinion, has been validated to date. The fact that a specific maneuver may be successful for a particular patient does not exclude the fact that all of these techniques are empiric and may be highly successful as performed by their proponents.

CHAPTER IV

INDICATIONS AND CONTRAINDICATIONS OF MANIPULATION

Indications

THE MOST FREQUENT indication for those who employ spinal manipulation is for so called functional low back pain. It is a non-specific diagnosis and it would appear to be the result of an acute trauma caused by excessive, inappropriate stress over the lumbosacral region. It is often associated with a history of a lateral rotational movement combined with flexion. Thus, excessive asymmetrical strain may be produced by unusual or sudden movement of the paravertebral musculature. Tenderness over the painful area is elicited. There is generally no radiation of pain nor localized neurological signs.

Other conditions where manipulation has been employed with some success include chronic low back pain, acute low back pain with a positive straight leg raising test, pain associated with a bulging intervertebral disc, piriformis syndrome, and posterior facet syndrome.

Contraindications

The contraindications to manipulation are manifold. They include any condition of the bone where there is fragility and potential instability from fractures, osteoporosis, osteomalacia, and osteogenesis imperfecta. These phenomena may be associated with other systemic conditions such as rheumatoid arthritis, metastatic bone disease due to malignancy, Paget's disease, and multiple myeloma. The presence of osteomylitis and progressive neurologic disease related to spinal cord pathology are conditions that mitigate against manipulation. Essentially any condition that may lead to spinal cord compression is an absolute contraindication for manipulative therapy.

Other medical conditions that are relative contraindications are based upon good clinical judgment and should be obvious to a qualified clinician. These include any bleeding diathesis, and the patient who is on anticoagulant therapy.

Complications

The perception of most lay people concerning musculoskeletal manipulation is that of a procedure which is safe and often efficaceous. To quote from a medical writer (Silk, 1982) in a county medical society journal, manipulation is considered a minor and essentially preventive form of healing. "Chiropractic survives because it is completely nonthreatening to the patient." Perhaps it is perceived that way, but in fact manipulation, when improperly or inappropriately applied, can have, on rare occasions, disastrous consequences.

As of 1980, Haldeman (1980) reports that there are less than 100 reported cases where serious complications of manipulative therapy have occurred. The severe complications arise from injury to the cerebral circulation or spinal cord due to cervical manipulation.

The most frequent complication of manipulation is the prolapse of a herniated intervertebral disc. Other complications include fracture of the odontoid process, atlanto-axial dislocation, cerebellar and brain stem trauma with thrombosis of vertebral, basilar and/or cerebellar arteries. Kewalramani et al (1982) have reported on myelopathy and myeloradiculopathy consequent to manipulation.

Deaths from manipulation have been reported in the literature. Krueger and Okazaki (1980) reported on one patient who died following a cervical manipulation with resultant vertebral basilar thrombosis. They provided reports on nine additional nonfatal cases. In addition, they reviewed 17 papers in the English literature describing 27 cases of similar pathology, bringing to a total of 37 reported cases of this complication. Five additional patients are described by Sherman et al (1981). It would appear that the majority of these 42 cases involve the atlanto-axial level. The mechanism of the lesion is presumably an interference of blood flow in the vertebro-basilar system during manipulation of the cervical spine sufficient to cause ischemia and subsequent infarction of the brain stem.

It is apparent that manipulation of the cervical spine has a potentially higher risk of serious complications than of the lumbar spine.

In Table IV-1 is a list of contraindications for manipulation. This list has been modified from Haldeman (1980).

Table IV-1

CONTRAINDICATIONS FOR MANIPULATION

Unstable fractures
Severe osteoporosis
Multiple myeloma
Osteomyelitis
Primary bone tumors
Metastatic bone tumors
Paget's disease
Any progressive neurological deficit
Spinal cord tumors
Cauda equina compression
Central intervertebral disc herniations
Hypermobile joints
Rheumatoid arthritis
Inflammatory phase of ankylosing spondylitis
Psoriatic arthritis
Reiter's syndrome
Anticoagulant therapy
Congenital bleeding disorders
Acquired bleeding disorders

Modified from Haldeman (1980)

In the light of these documented reports, the contraindications should not be taken lightly. It is true that these reports reflect a minute proportion of the millions of manipulations that have been performed in the English-speaking world. However, those that are reported are sufficiently dangerous to warrant caution. Furthermore, it is likely that there are numerous patients whose spinal cord or brain have been temporarily compromised with momentary and reversible symptoms that have gone unreported. All those—be they osteopathic or allopathic physician, chiropractor or physical therapist—who would manipulate the spine should take heed.

On the other hand, one might consider the dangers of other interventions for low back pain. For example, surgery for a herniated disc may lead to nerve damage, wound infection, excessive bleeding with its implied dangers, and postoperative arachnoiditis and adhesions.

In an interesting controlled study with a ten-year follow-up of surgery performed for herniated disc, Weber found a statistically significant better result for the surgically treated group, one year after. That is, the results of surgery were significantly better than conservative therapy. However, comparison of the results after four years did not show a statistically significant difference, although the tendency to a more favorable effect of surgery was retained. This tendency persisted even after nine years of follow-up.

In the nonoperated group approximately 61% of the patients were either cured or showed satisfactory improvement. Weber therefore suggests that approximately 60% of the operated patients may have been submitted to an unnecessary surgical procedure. Many of these patients perhaps might have been relieved by manipulation therapy.

Injection of the painful area or joint with a steroid and an anesthetic may lead to a hypersensitivity or anaphylactic response. Trauma to the tissues and inadvertant bleeding may result. Chemonucleolysis is one type of injection employing chymopapain. This substance may rarely lead to death due to anaphylactic reaction. Because of this risk a repeat injection of chymopapain is contraindicated.

CHAPTER V

GUIDELINES FOR VALID CONTROLLED CLINICAL TRIALS

ALTHOUGH there have been numerous reports indicating the efficacy of spinal manipulation (e.g. Chrisman et al, 1964; Ware, 1972), very few controlled clinical trials have been performed. Anecdotal evidence or data from a series of treated patients are often useful. However, this type of evidence can also be quite misleading. With many diseases, some proportion of the patients can be expected to improve regardless of the treatment employed. In the case of back pain, this proportion may be very high. According to Nachemson (1976) 70% of back pain patients get well within three weeks and 90% get well within three months regardless of the nature of the treatment.

A further problem for the evaluation of treatment, is the placebo effect. The therapeutic effect may result simply from the patient's or the physician's belief in the treatment's efficacy. The method of randomized clinical trials was developed to assess and control for the placebo effect and any other factors that might bias the results.

Randomized clinical trials are designed to prevent the appearance of conscious or unconscious bias at every step of the study as follows:

1. The first step involves the careful selection of patients for the study. Patients can only be admitted to the study if they meet the entrance criterion and if the physician is willing to treat them using any of the therapies under investigation. The physician should *not* admit patients to the study and then remove them if the treatment they are scheduled to receive does not seem appropriate. It is extremely important that the individual admitting patients to the trial does not know which treatment those patients will receive if they are admitted.

2. The next stage is the assignment of patients to the treatments under investigation. These will include one or more active therapies and usually, a control treatment believed to be equivalent to no effective therapy. Assignment to treatments must be random. The simplest procedure is to simply toss a coin and assign the patient on that basis. However, this procedure, and its more complex analogs involving computerized random number generators, cannot guarantee the number of patients assigned to each group and, in small studies, these numbers may be grossly unequal. A more common procedure is to maintain a supply of opaque sealed envelopes containing the name of the group to which an individual patient will be assigned. When the patient is selected for the study, the envelope will be opened and the patient will be assigned to the group indicated. Using this method it is possible to precisely control the numbers of patients assigned to each treatment group.

   There is some disagreement over whether or not groups should be stratified. Stratification is an attempt to reduce the random variance between groups. For example, a study stratified by sex might require 50 males and 50 females, 25 of each to receive the experimental treatment while the remaining 25 receive the control treatment. Essentially, this would require two separate boxes of sealed envelopes. Stratification is scientifically desirable and is recommended by Greenland et al (1980), but it is obvious that not many variables can be controlled in this fashion. For example, stratification based on sex, three levels of age, and three stages of disease would require $2 \times 3 \times 3 = 18$ separate boxes of sealed envelopes. We tend to agree with Peto et al (1976), that administrative problems of stratification usually outweigh its statistical advantages and we recommend its use only in the case of variables that are known to be highly correlated with the outcome of treatment. For example, treatment of chronic back pain is usually less successful than treatment of acute back pain (e.g. Hoehler and Tobis, 1983) and it would, therefore, be useful to include an equivalent number of chronic pain patients in the treated and control groups.
3. The next stage involves the application of the various therapies to the patients. In the "ideal" type of clinical trial—the double-blind placebo-controlled experiment—neither the patient nor the physician is aware of the nature of the treatment received. In drug studies, this is accomplished through the use of a placebo tablet or injection designed to mimic the appearance of the actual drug un-

der investigation. In studies of many non-drug therapies, a true placebo control is impossible. However, it is still desirable to minimize the patient's exposure to information indicating the expected outcome of the clinical trial.

4. Conceptually, the final stage of a clinical trial is the assessment of the results although assessments will of course occur throughout the treatment process in a study of any protracted therapy. In order for valid results to be obtained, the individual making the assessment must not be given any indication of the treatment received. This is especially important if the response to treatment is "subjective" for example, reduced pain.

A clinical trial of spinal manipulation will face special problems at each of the above stages.

1. At the stage of patient selection, it will be handicapped by the absence of any generally accepted diagnostic criteria defining patients who are appropriate for manipulative therapy. Diagnosis is fundamentally subjective, primarily involving musculoskeletal palpation rather than objective laboratory measurements. Furthermore, there is considerable disagreement between the various theoretical schools of manipulation and there has been little success in resolving these differences through experimental research.
2. Because the factors predicting the success of manipulation therapy are largely unknown it is virtually impossible to stratify patients in any meaningful way. It is also difficult to account for the variability of response using post hoc statistical analyses. This lack of knowledge regarding prognostic factors in spinal manipulation insures that there will be a large amount of residual variability in the response to treatment. This excess variability will tend to cloud any assessment of the results of the clinical trial.
3. There is considerable disagreement regarding the appropriate manipulative therapy to employ. We have discussed the various types of manipulation favored by the various theoretical schools. In addition, the exact form of manipulative treatment employed will depend on each individual clinician's assessment of each individual patient. This source of variability can be reduced but only at the cost of greatly reducing the generality of the results. For example, a clinical trial in which all treatment was delivered by one osteopathically trained physician, might be characterized by a highly

consistent treatment methodology but it might also produce results that would be valid only for osteopathic physicians or, worse, valid only for the particular osteopathic physician employed in the trial.

An even more serious problem is the difficulty involved in the design of an appropriate control group. A placebo control, similar to that used in drug studies, can not be used because the physician will always be aware of the treatment that he is delivering and the patient will not be easily deceived. A typical control has involved the use of such treatments as oral analgesics (Evans et al, 1978) or shortwave diathermy (Glover et al, 1974). This is clearly unsatisfactory because these treatments do not involve any manual interaction between patient and physician and hence cannot control for the effect of "laying on of hands." This effect might easily produce a spurious superiority of manipulative therapy if an equivalently enthusiastic "laying on of hands" is not provided for the control group as well.

4. The impossibility of a true placebo control must also affect the final assessment of the results of treatment. Bias can be largely prevented if the clinician making the assessment is not aware of the nature of the treatment each patient has received. However, if the patient is aware of the nature of his or her treatment that awareness may, somehow, be communicated to the assessor. Furthermore, if the measure of therapeutic success is subjective—i.e. the alleviation of "pain"—the patient is, in effect, responsible for the assessment of the results of treatment.

Measurement of Back Pain

One of the major difficulties in studies of manipulative treatments for back pain is the lack of any generally recognized measure of the extent or type of pathology responsible for the subjective complaint. In the absence of valid and reliable measures, both diagnosis and assessment of the success of therapy must necessarily involve the subjective impressions of either the physician or the patient. Thus, clinical trials of spinal manipulation must typically rely on subjective measures of treatment efficacy in unblinded studies performed on poorly characterized patient populations. For this reason, clinical trials of manipulation have been difficult to conduct and have been viewed with some skepticism by the scientific community. Apart from its importance in scientific investigations, adequate measurement will be necessary if manipulative treatments are ever to be systematically applied in an appropriate fashion to appropriate patients. Methods that are currently in use or contemplated for the future are described below.

Subjective Reduction in Pain or Other Symptoms

Despite the difficulties in interpretation, most clinical trials of spinal manipulation have relied heavily on subjective measures of back pain. Glover et al (1974), requested patients to assess the amount of relief from pain on a scale of 0 to 100. Manipulation was significantly better than control treatments only immediately after treatment in a subgroup of patients with a first attack of acute back pain. Doran and Newell (1975) requested both the patient and the physician to assess level of pain on a six-point scale of "worse," "unchanged," "slightly improved," "moderately improved," "markedly improved," and "completely relieved." Data were collected after the three-week course of treatment and later at six weeks and three months from the initial examination. The three month follow-up was done by mail and had a relatively high (73%) response rate. As the data were originally analyzed (using chi-square tests), no significant differences were observed, but a recent re-analysis using more appropriate statistical methods (Greenland, et al, 1980) found that patients treated by spinal manipulation reported significantly more relief at three weeks. The level of correlation between the subjective responses of patients and physicians was not reported although it was claimed that "patients' assessments concurred closely with those of the doctor."

Evans et al (1978), used a four point scale of 0 = nil, 1 = mild, 2 = moderate, 3 = severe. At the end of each treatment period, patients assessed the efficacy of treatment using the scale, ineffective, equivocal, effective, or highly effective. Subjective pain assessments were verified by monitoring the number of codeine phosphate capsules consumed (patients had been instructed to take the capsules only as necessary to control pain). The two measures were highly correlated ($r = 0.92$, $p = .001$). Small positive effects of manipulation were observed but the statistical methods used were not adequate to determine the reliability of this effect.

In the studies by Jayson et al (1981), subjective levels of pain were scored on a six-point scale of much worse, slightly worse, no change, slightly better, much better, or completely better. Global assessment of the efficacy of therapy was rated as, made it worse, useless, some help, very helpful. General level of activity was scored as unable to work, restricted activity or completely normal. None of these measures showed any significant effect due to spinal manipulation.

Hoehler et al (1981) used subjective measures of relief of pain on a scale of much worse, somewhat worse, no change, somewhat better, or much better. A wide variety of indicators of flexibility and range of motion (walking, bending, sitting down in a chair, sitting up in bed, reaching and dressing) were subjectively assessed on a three point scale, worse, no change or improved. Most of these measures yielded significant differences between manipulated and control patients immediately after treatment.

An unusual use of subjective measures was reported by Fisk (1977a) who requested patients to assess their level of pain every few hours for a period of several days. Thus, it was possible to obtain information concerning the temporal characteristics of the pain relief produced by spinal manipulation. For example, it was possible to identify a subset of patients who, although they experienced immediate relief, showed a rapid return of symptoms—sometimes within several hours of the manipulative treatment.

In a similar study, we used the above mentioned five-point pain scale ranging from 1 (much better) to 5 (much worse). Subjective pain scores over a period of up to four days after manipulation are shown in Table V-1.

Patients with chronic and acute back pain experience equivalent immediate relief from pain but, in chronic back pain patients, the symptoms tend to return. Subjective measures have been extensively used in studies of spinal manipulation. These can provide much useful information but, because of the impossibility of fully blinding clinical trials of

Table V-1

PAIN SCORES AFTER MANIPULATION

	MALES		FEMALES	
	ACUTE N = 21	CHRONIC N = 13	ACUTE N = 9	CHRONIC N = 18
IMMEDIATE	1.95	2.15	1.67	1.89
1 HOUR	2.14	2.23	1.44	2.06
4 HOURS	2.33	2.23	2.00	2.06
1 DAY	2.00	2.92	2.33	2.94
4 DAYS	1.90	3.15	2.33	3.28

manual therapy and the high likelihood of placebo effects, these studies have not been entirely convincing. For this reason, there have been numerous attempts to develop relatively objective measures of back pain.

Changes in Posture or Range of Motion

Goniometric or other measurements of posture and range of motion have been quite popular as measures of the pathophysiologic processes underlying back pain. These measures have generally been found to be relatively consistent (Lankhorst et al, 1982) and generally correlated with clinical diagnosis of back pain (Meyer et al, 1984) although negative results have been reported (Sweetman et al, 1974).

The classic range-of-motion test used in the assessment of back pain is Lassegue's sign of restriction in straight leg raising (see Figure VI-1). When the knee is extended, raising the leg more than 30° puts traction on the sciatic nerve which will, presumably, produce severe pain in a patient with a disc herniation impinging on the nerve root. However, the unique relationship between straight leg raising and disc involvement has recently been questioned and the straight leg raising test is now

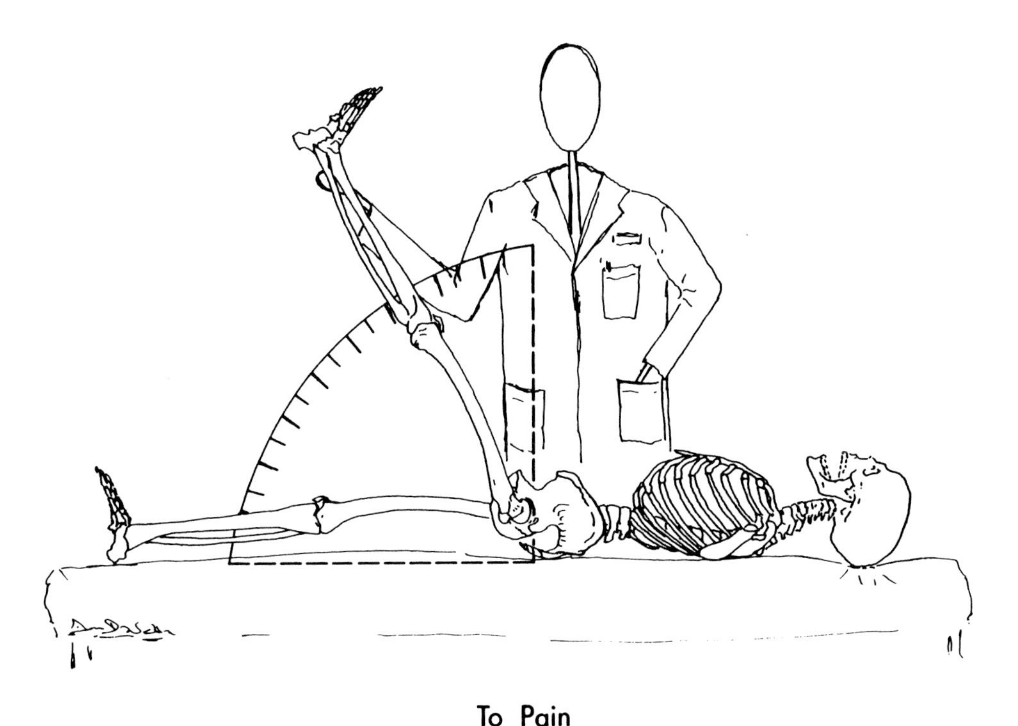

Figure V-1. The straight-leg raising test with pain as the endpoint.

thought to be, primarily, a test of spasm of the paraspinal, gluteal and hamstring muscles (Fisk, 1975).

An early uncontrolled study by Chrisman et al (1964), as well as the more recent one by Fisk (1975), have shown that spinal manipulation is usually followed by increases in the angle of straight leg raising. Further studies have elaborated variations of the straight leg raising test specifically designed to measure hamstring stretch. One of these is a test commonly used by osteopathic physicians (Moran et al, 1973) in which the palm of one hand is placed over the contralateral anterior superior iliac spine and the leg is raised with the other hand until pelvic rotation is palpable (see Figure V-2). Fisk (1979a) trained physiotherapists to perform this test and demonstrated a high degree of reliability, when different examiners tested the same subject. Measurements utilizing a tension gauge were even more reliable. In a controlled clinical trial, it was demonstrated that selected patients with unilateral low back pain show substantial decreases in hamstring tightness as a result of spinal manipulation (Fisk, 1979b). Other studies have indicated that low back pain is characterized by a significant difference between the right and left sides and this difference is eliminated by spinal manipulation (Fisk, 1977a).

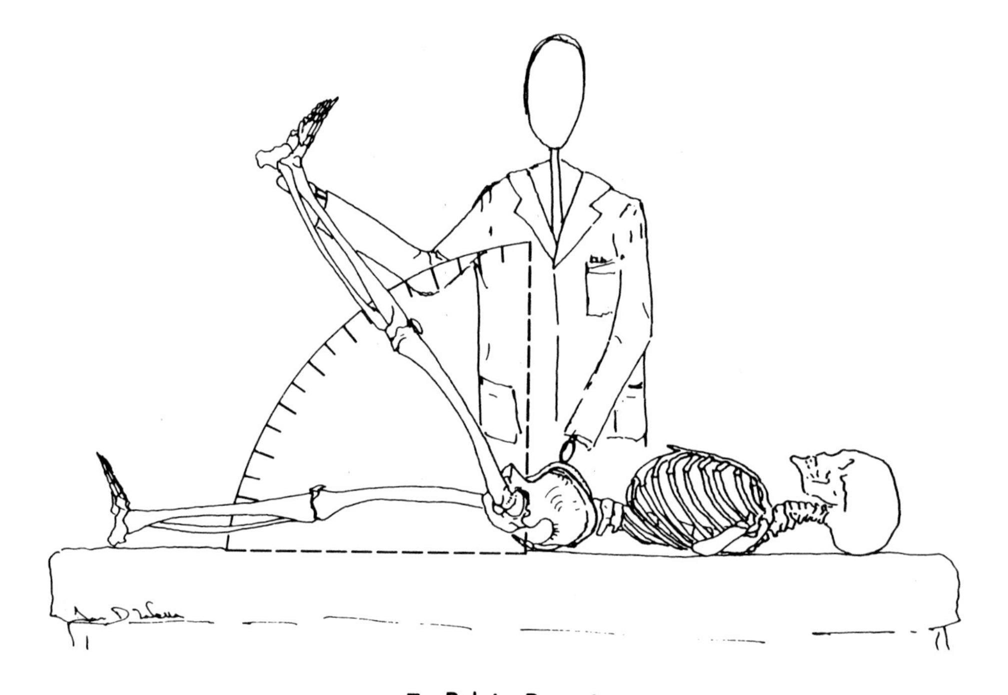

Figure V-2. The straight-leg raising test with pelvic rotation as the endpoint.

The classic straight leg raising test has been employed in several recent controlled clinical trials. Jayson et al (1981) examined a group of 87 patients of general practitioners and 92 hospital patients given either Maitland's (1977) mobilization manipulation techniques, or placebo microwave diathermy. After one month of treatment, manipulated patients showed significant increase in the angle of straight-leg raising while control patients showed no change. However, because the manipulated patients had lower pre-treatment levels of straight-leg raising, differences between groups were not statistically significant. In this study, mean angles of straight leg raising were 68°-76° prior to treatment. Similar initial levels were observed by Hoehler et al (1981) and Farrell and Twomey (1982). Hoehler et al (1981) reported relatively small but significant increases in straight leg raising due to spinal manipulation while Farrell and Twomey (1982) reported no significant effect. In contrast, Nwuga (1982) conducted a controlled clinical trial in which all patients had acute low back pain attributed to disc protrusion. As might be expected, these patients had severe restriction of straight leg raising prior to treatment (29°-31°) and displayed substantial differences afterwards. Angle of straight leg raising increased to 68° in the manipulated patients and remained at 35° in the controls.

The two different straight-leg raising tests were compared in studies by Hoehler et al (1981) and Hoehler and Tobis (1982). In a controlled clinical trial, it was shown that the classic straight-leg-raising test yielded a small immediate increase in the manipulated patients (3.3°) and no change (-0.5°) in the controls. This difference was statistically significant. However, by the end of treatment, the manipulated and control groups showed similar improvement (Hoehler et al, 1981). Using the Fisk (1975) test of hamstring tightness, there was no immediate difference, although at the end of treatment, a small non-significant difference was observed (manipulated: 8.0°; control: 4.1°). In a study of interexaminer reliability, Hoehler and Tobis (1982) found that the classic straight leg raising test was far more reliable and was more likely to distinguish low back pain patients from those without low back pain. However, both straight-leg raising tests were significantly improved by spinal manipulation. It was suggested that, if Fisk's (1975) hamstring tightness test is to be used in studies of back pain, the investigators must pay careful attention to problems of interexaminer reliability.

Another commonly used measure involves the assessment of forward flexion. The method used is generally based on Schober's (1937) test, or a modification of that test described by Macrae and Wright (1969). Flexion is measured by the increase in the distance between marks made on the skin over the lumbosacral spine. In a crossover study, Evans et al (1978) found significant increases in forward flexion during periods in which patients were being treated by spinal manipulation. In another clinical trial, Rasmussen (1979) reported that all 12 manipulated patients showed increased forward flexion, while only 6 of 12 controls showed any improvement. Increased mobility in manipulated patients was also reported by Nwuga (1982) who measured flexion and extension using a spondylometer. However, Farrell and Twomey (1982) using the same instrument and Jayson et al (1981) using a goniometer found no effects of manipulation on forward flexion. Another measure of forward flexion is the distance from the fingers to the floor during maximal forward bending. Two clinical trials using this measurement failed to observe any effect of spinal manipulation (Doran and Newell, 1975; Hoehler et al, 1981). A recent study that investigated a number of measures of spinal flexibility found that, while anterior flexion was diminished in patients with low back pain and could be scored with a fairly high degree of reliability it did not appear to be greatly affected by spinal manipulation (Hoehler and Tobis, 1982).

As noted above, Nwuga (1982) apparently found significant effects of manipulation on extension. He also reported significant increase in lateral flexion and rotation. However, Farrell and Twomey (1982) reported significant improvement in extension, but not rotation, and Jayson et al (1981) reported no effects on either extension or lateral flexion.

A wide variety of tests of spinal flexibility and postural asymmetry were investigated by Hoehler and Tobis (1982). All patients received the following tests:

1. Scapular asymmetry as measured (in degrees) with the patient standing, from marks placed on the inferior angles of the scapula.
2. Pelvic asymmetry as measured (in degrees) with the patient standing, from marks placed on the iliac crests.
3. Left and right lateral bending as measured in degrees of arc between the true vertical and a line extending from S1 to T7.
4. Anterior spinal flexion measured in centimetres using the method of Macrae and Wright (1969).
5. Asymmetry of malleolar levels (in cm) measured with the patient supine as described by Moran et al (1973). This is a measure of functional inequality of leg length.

6. Eversion of the feet measured in degrees of arc between the true vertical and the resting angle of the foot, with the patient supine. This test has been used as an indicator of piriformis spasm (Retzloff et al, 1974).
7. Hamstring tightness using the modification of the straight leg raising test described by Moran et al (1973) and Fisk (1975). This test requires the examiner to raise the patient's leg until motion is palpated in the contralateral pelvic crest.
8. Passive straight leg raising to pain.
9. Voluntary straight leg raising to pain.

Table V-2

OBJECTIVE MEASURES IN PATIENTS WITH AND WITHOUT LOW BACK PAIN

	With low back pain Mean (SD)	Without low back pain Mean (SD)	t
Tests of flexibility:			
Anterior flexion (cm)	5.5 (1.8)	7.8 (2.5)	2.70*
Lateral flexion	23 (8)	30 (11)	1.83
Hamstring tightness	56 (10)	61 (6)	1.18
Passive SLR	65 (15)	77 (7)	2.29*
Voluntary SLR	63 (21)	79 (7)	2.20*
Foot eversion	45 (11)	44 (18)	0.17
Tests of asymmetry:			
Lateral flexion	3.7 (2.7)	3.4 (2.4)	0.31
Hamstring tightness	3.0 (3.0)	2.1 (1.3)	0.76
Passive SLR	4.8 (2.8)	3.5 (2.5)	1.19
Voluntary SLR	4.5 (6.0)	4.0 (6.2)	0.19
Foot eversion	6.9 (4.4)	3.3 (2.9)	2.15*
Malleolar levels (cm)	0.33(0.31)	0.24(0.19)	0.71
Iliac levels	1.6 (1.3)	1.3 (1.2)	0.74
Scapular levels	1.8 (1.6)	2.3 (2.6)	0.58

Measures are in degrees unless otherwise noted.
*$p < 0.05$

From Hoehler and Tobis (1982)

Each test was repeated by two independent examiners. If manipulative treatment was warranted, it was given and the tests were repeated for the third time.

Note that these measures may be divided into two broad categories, those which test for asymmetry and those which test for flexibility. The foot eversion measure is a special case in that it tests the resting state of internal and external rotators. With the exception of anterior flexion, all measures of flexibility can also yield a measure of asymmetry by taking the absolute value of the difference between the right and left sides.

Table V-2 compares patients with low back pain vs. patients with thoracic or shoulder pain (but no low back pain) using the means of the pretreatment scores obtained by the two examiners.

Table V-3

RELIABILITY OF THE OBJECTIVE MEASURES

	Mean absolute error (degrees or cm)	Standard score of absolute error	r
Tests of flexibility:			
Anterior flexion	1.7	0.66	0.50**
Lateral flexion	5.6	0.55	0.71**
Hamstring tightness	9.0	0.97	0.36*
Passive SLR	8.0	0.52	0.78**
Voluntary SLR	4.7	0.24	0.95**
Foot eversion	9.9	0.77	0.63**
Tests of asymmetry:			
Lateral flexion	4.4	0.78	0.23
Hamstring tightness	3.4	0.67	-0.04
Passive SLR	6.0	0.99	0.32
Active SLR	3.5	0.41	0.44*
Foot eversion	5.0	0.63	0.38*
Malleolar levels	0.35	0.79	0.33
Iliac levels	1.9	0.89	0.37*
Scapular levels	2.5	0.91	0.43*

*$p < 0.05$;P < 0.01

From Hoehler and Tobis (1982)

Table V-3 shows measures of agreement for each of the objective measures. The first column shows the means of the absolute values of the differences between the first and second examination. The second column shows standard scores based on the mean absolute error divided by the geometric mean of the standard deviations obtained from the first and the second examination. High levels of reliability are indicated by a low standard score. The third column shows the Pearson r coefficient of correlation between the first and the second examination. Perfect correlation would be indicated by a value of 1.00 while the complete absence of any correlation would be indicated by a value of zero.

Table V-4 shows pretreatment and post-treatment measures in the eight subjects who reported relief of pain after spinal manipulation.

Table V-4

OBJECTIVE MEASURES BEFORE AND AFTER TREATMENT

	Pre-Treatment Mean (SD)	Post-Treatment Mean (SD)	t
Tests of flexibility:			
Anterior flexion (cm)	6.8 (1.4)	7.1 (1.5)	0.55
Lateral flexion	25 (9)	26 (11)	0.38
Hamstring tightness	52 (8)	57 (10)	3.95**
Passive SLR	69 (10)	74 (10)	3.69**
Voluntary SLR	69 (13)	73 (12)	3.59**
Foot eversion	50 (9)	50 (11)	0.08
Tests of asymmetry:			
Lateral flexion	5.0 (3.7)	6.5 (7.5)	0.52
Hamstring tightness	5.0 (3.1)	3.1 (2.8)	1.56
Passive SLR	8.4 (5.0)	5.9 (6.0)	1.85
Voluntary SLR	6.3 (4.2)	2.3 (2.1)	3.35**
Foot eversion	10.4 (4.5)	10.6 (6.9)	0.13
Malleolar levels (cm)	0.25(0.38)	0.06(0.18)	1.43
Iliac levels	2.0 (1.9)	2.0 (1.8)	0.00
Scapular levels	2.6 (2.3)	2.0 (2.1)	1.67

Measures are in degrees unless otherwise noted.
$^{*}p < 0.05$; $^{**}p < 0.01$

From Hoehler and Tobis (1982)

For a test to be useful in clinical investigations of spinal manipulation, it must be valid. That is, it must be correlated with the presence or absence of low back pain (see Table V-2). Furthermore, it should be reliable. That is, in the absence of treatment, patients should not show major changes between re-examinations (see Table V-2). Finally, the test should measure the effects produced by spinal manipulation (see Table V-4). Of the measures examined here, only straight leg raising meets all three criteria.

Radiography

If one agrees with the chiropractors that manipulation produces its effects through the "adjustment" of displaced vertebrae, or if one agrees with Cyriax (1971, 1982) that the beneficial effects of manipulation result from displacement of fragments of a disc, radiography would appear to be a useful means of objectively documenting the effects of treatment. Indeed, Mathews and Yates (1969) observed reduction in a prolapsed disc following a successful spinal manipulation. However, systematic radiographic studies conducted during controlled clinical trials have found no effects attributable to spinal manipulation (Roberts et al, 1978).

With the high resolution that has been more recently achieved with computerized axial tomography (CAT) scanners (e.g. Bell et al, 1984), the possibility exists that small morphological changes may yet be observed following intervention by manipulation.

Electromyography

Electrophysiological testing has long been used in the examination of back pain patients—primarily in the investigation of the effects of nerve root compression on the latency of spinal reflexes. Malcolm (1951) was among the first to report slowing of knee and ankle jerk responses in sciatica and other lumbar and sacral root compression syndromes. More recently, investigators have used the Hoffman (H) reflex—an electrically induced analog of the ankle jerk—to study the effects of lumbosacral disc herniation on spinal reflexes. In true nerve root compression syndromes, the latency of the H reflex is invariably increased (Braddom and Johnson, 1974; Deschuytere and Rosselle, 1970; Fisher et al, 1978; Kamihira, 1968; Schuchman, 1978).

The relevance of reflex latency tests to spinal manipulation is questionable. However, if, as proposed by Cyriax (1966), manipulation achieves its results by dislodging fragments on a herniated disc, one might expect to observe changes in the latency of spinal reflexes following treatment. A recent study by Hoehler and Buerger (1981), tested H reflexes of six low back pain patients before and after spinal manipulation therapy. No consistent changes in either reflex latency or reflex amplitude were observed. However, because of the small number of patients tested and because testing was only carried out immediately after treatment, these results do not constitute strong evidence against an effect of manipulation on spinal reflexes.

Direct recording from areas of "osteopathic" lesions were first attempted by Denslow and Hassett (1942) who reported spontaneous spike activity in areas of palpable tenderness. Similar findings were reported in patients with sciatica by Elliott (1944) and after musculoskeletal disorders by Arroyo (1966). In contrast, Kraft et al (1968) reported electrical silence in muscle spasm but it is possible that this may have been due to an insufficiently sensitive recording technique (Cobb et al, 1975).

De Vries (1968, Cobb et al, 1975) has reported several studies in which EMG levels in sore muscles directly paralleled the extent of muscle soreness over a period of time. However, a more recent study of artificially induced muscle soreness found a dissociation between EMG levels and pain (McGlynn, 1975). EMG biofeedback or muscle stretching produced substantial differences in EMG levels without any significant effect on subjectively experienced levels of pain.

If it is presumed that increased paraspinal muscle tension is associated with back pain, the back pain patients should display elevated paraspinal surface EMG levels, and these elevations should be decreased by a successful treatment. However, studies reported by different investigators have produced apparently contradictory results. Paraspinal EMG amplitudes in back pain patients have been reported to be both elevated (Hoyt et al, 1981) and depressed (Collins et al, 1982). Bobinac-Georgievski and Muftic (1981) reported that, as compared to controls, back pain patients had higher EMG activity during forward bending and lower EMG activity during backward bending. Kravitz et al (1981) found that back pain patients have higher paraspinal EMG levels than controls only when attempting to relax the paraspinal muscles while contracting other muscle groups. Soderberg and Barr (1983) reported that back-pain patients had elevated EMG levels while standing but, during various activities that produced increased EMG levels in normal controls, back-pain patients showed little or no change. The variable of time was investigated by Jayasinghe et al (1978) who reported that low back pain patients showed increasing EMG activity while standing quietly for six minutes. Controls showed a decrease in EMG activity. De Vries (1968) reported similar effects and found that increasing EMG levels were correlated with the appearance of pain.

Studies of the effects of treatment for low back pain are equally confusing. Brena et al (1980) reported no change in EMG activity after lumbar sympathetic blocks despite the findings of pain relief. Basmajian (1978) found an increase in paraspinal EMG activity following successful treatment for low back pain.

We have recently examined the effects of spinal manipulation on EMGs of patients with unilateral low back pain. Paraspinal surface EMG activity was recorded during a six minute period before and after treatment. As shown in Table V-5 relative electromyographic activity was substantially lower on the painful side. This difference may reflect minor postural adjustments necessary to maintain balance. It is not surprising that, during an episode of low back pain, the painful side would be less likely to participate in such postural adjustment. On average, spinal manipulation produced a slight reduction in electromyographic activity on the nonpainful side. This reduction was more remarkable in several individual patients. An example is shown in Figure V-3. However, as in the H reflex study, only a small number of patients were observed and only the immediate effects of manipulation were assessed. Electromyographic measures of the effects of manipulation would seem to be potentially useful but, they have never been adequately investigated (Nouwen and Bush, 1984).

Table V-5

RELATIVE EMG ACTIVITY BEFORE AND AFTER SPINAL MANIPULATION

	Painful Side Mean (SD)	Nonpainful Side Mean (SD)
Pre-treatment (N = 8)		
First half of session	0.91 (0.14)	1.11 (0.15)
Second half of session	0.85 (0.11)	1.13 (0.11)
Post-treatment (N = 8)		
First half of session	0.87 (0.20)	1.12 (0.12)
Second half of session	0.85 (0.20)	1.01 (0.13)

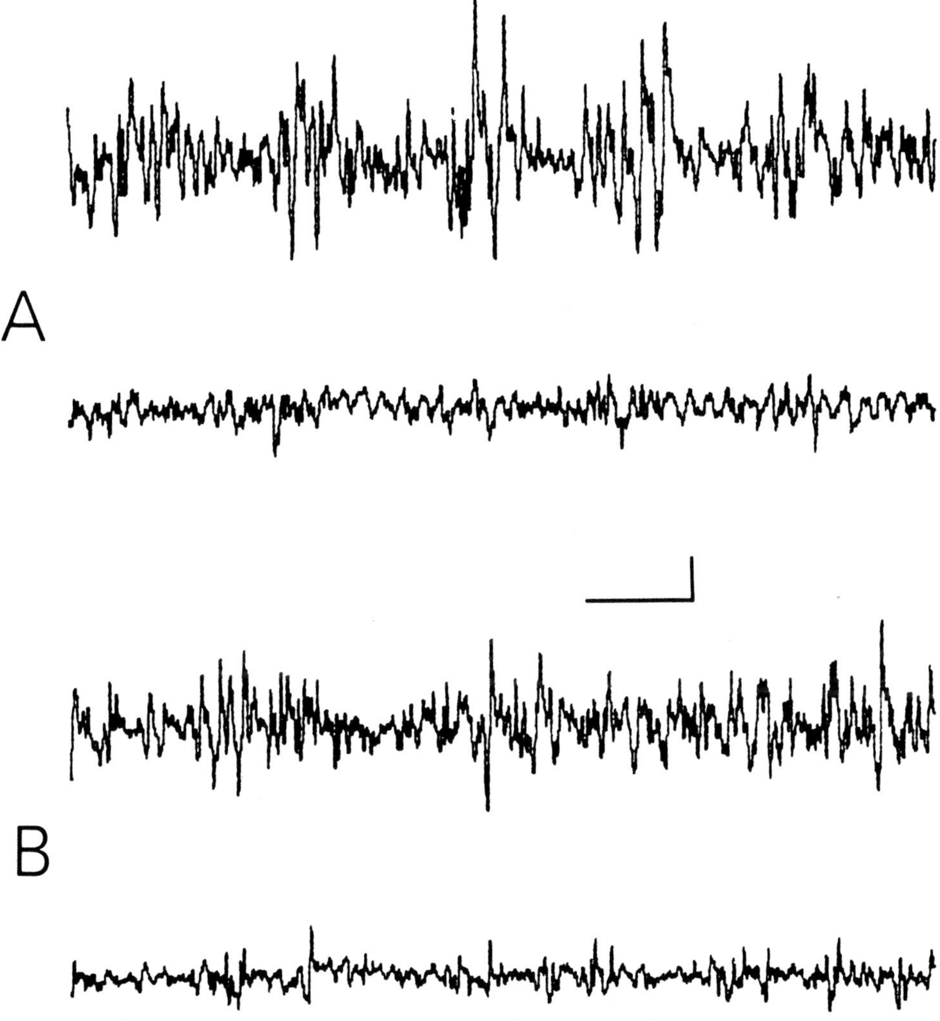

Figure V-3. EMG recordings from a patient who showed effects of spinal manipulation. A: Before manipulation. B: After manipulation. The upper tracings are from the nonpainful side, while the lower tracings are from the painful side. Calibration marks: 100 msec and 1 mV.

Electrical Skin Resistance

Another biomedical measure that has been used is the investigation of myofascial pain as electrical resistance of the skin. Korr et al (1962) showed that injection of hypertonic saline into the paraspinal tissues produced areas of lowered electrical resistance. A later study reported similar findings in naturally occuring musculoskeletal disturbances and pain syndromes (Korr, et al, 1964). However, electrical skin resistance is not a highly reliable measure and has received little recent attention.

Thermography

Infrared thermography was first investigated in back pain patients by Albert et al (1964), Goldberg et al (1964), and Edeiken et al (1968) who used it to localize herniated discs. Abnormal thermograms were also reported in ankylosing spondylitis (Agarwall et al, 1970). More recently, a cheaper method—liquid crystal thermography—has also been found to be useful in the study of herniated discs (Pochaczevsky, 1983) and the demonstration of soft tissue lesions associated with nonspecific low back pain (Rubal, 1982; Tichauer, 1977).

Palpation

The above techniques are essentially methods of objectively analyzing and quantifying the variables which the typical practitioner of manipulative medicine observes through diagnostic palpation. Although palpation is extensively used, it has not received much study. Several investigators have demonstrated correlations between back pain syndromes and cutaneous hyperesthesia or tenderness (Glover, 1970; Gunn et al, 1976, 1978).

Most work, however, has appeared in the osteopathic literature. Adams et al (1982) have recently discussed the importance of thermal

Table V-6

RELATIONSHIP BETWEEN THE PHYSICIAN'S IMPRESSION OF THE PATIENT'S SUSCEPTIBILITY TO MANIPULATION AND THE PATIENT'S SUBJECTIVE RESPONSE TO MANIPULATIVE THERAPY

		PHYSICIAN'S PREDICTED BENEFIT OF MANIPULATION			
		Very Good	Good	Fair	Poor
PATIENT'S	Much Better	51	38	42	6
ASSESSMENT	Somewhat Better	37	41	31	5
OF RSULTS	No Change	6	6	19	4
OF MANIPU-	Somewhat Worse	1	1	1	1
LATION	Much Worse	0	0	0	0

From Buerger (1980)

sensitivity in palpation and, in a series of studies Johnston et al (1978, 1982a, 1982b) and Beal et al (1980) have attempted to determine the reliability of palpatory diagnosis and the stability of palpatory cues. The results have not, as yet, been particularly encouraging. Palpatory cues appear to be quite unstable and strong agreement between examiners is only seen in selected subjects.

The prognostic value of palpatory cues has been investigated by Buerger (1980) who collected data from a clinical trial of spinal manipulation for low back pain and correlated the physician's prediction (based largely on palpation) of the likelihood that the patient would benefit from manipulation and the patient's assessment of the actual benefit of that treatment. As shown in Table V-6, there was a positive correlation that was statistically significant ($p < .01$), but not particularly large ($r = .137$).

CHAPTER VI

RESULTS OF CLINICAL TRIALS OF SPINAL MANIPULATION

Coyer and Curwen

AN EARLY clinical trial of spinal manipulation was reported by Coyer and Curwen (1955). In this study, low back pain patients were alternately assigned to either manipulative treatment using the methods described by Cyriax (1971, 1982) or bedrest and analgesics. Thus, two groups of 76 patients each were entered into the study. Apparently, 16 of the patients in the control group dropped out of the study. In contrast, no patient dropped out of the manipulated group. At one week, 50% of the manipulated patients and only 27% of the control patients had recovered. At six weeks recovery was reported by 88% of the manipulated patients and 72% of the control patients. "Recovery" was not clearly defined and was, apparently, not assessed in a blinded fashion. Furthermore, the study was not truly randomized. Despite these deficits, this clinical trial suggests a substantial and significant beneficial effect of spinal manipulation.

Glover et al

The first truly randomized controlled clinical trial of spinal manipulation to be reported in the English-language medical literature was conducted by Glover, Morris and Khosla (1974). The patients were 84 employees reporting to an engineering works medical center with unilateral low back pain. Treated patients received a single rotational manipulation of the lumbosacral region. The primary response variable was the patient's subjective impression of relief from pain rated on a scale of 0 to 100. Figure VI-1, shows the results for all patients, while

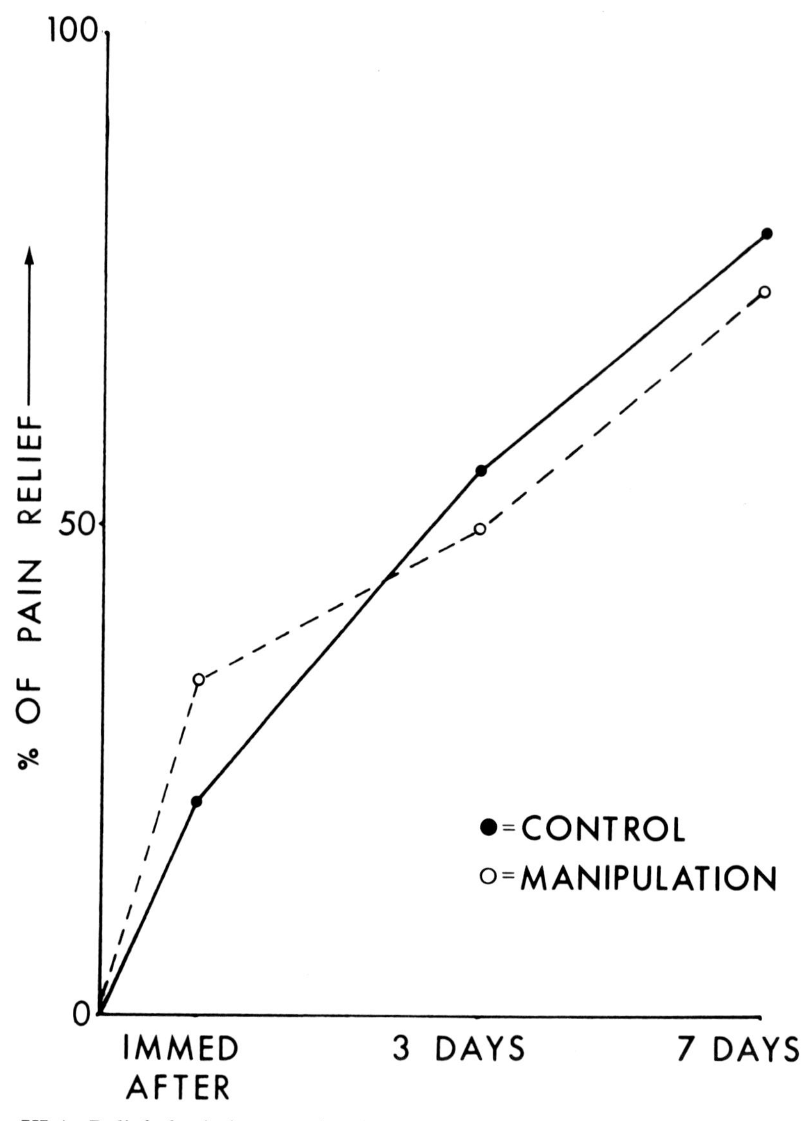

Figure VI-1. Relief of pain in control and manipulated groups (from Glover et al, 1974).

Figure VI-2 shows the results for the subgroup of patients with "acute" low back pain (duration less than 7 days). Manipulation produced significantly more relief in the "acute" patients but this difference was only apparent immediately after treatment. No differences were seen when patients were reexamined three or seven days later. Thus, some effect of manipulation was demonstrated but only in the subgroup of patients with acute low back pain. However, this conclusion is weakened by the absence of an adequate control group (simulated diathermy is little different from no treatment at all), and by the subjective nature of the measure of treatment efficacy. Furthermore, this was a trial of the manipulative techniques of only one clinician (the senior author) and, therefore, it may not be generally applicable.

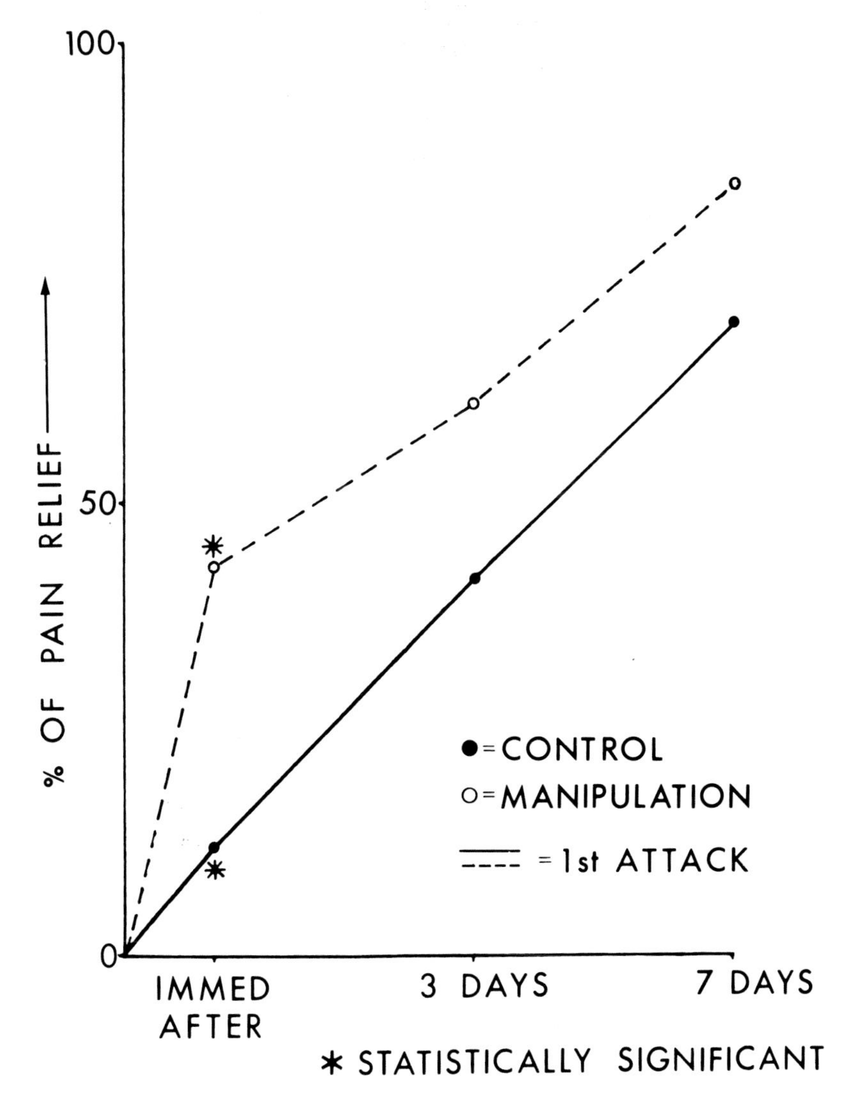

Figure VI-2. Relief of pain in patients in their first attack which lasted less than seven days at the time of treatment (from Glover et al, 1974).

Doran and Newell

Perhaps the most extensive study of manipulation was a multicenter clinical trial reported by Doran and Newell (1975). In this study, a total of 456 patients were treated at 7 separate centers. Treatments employed were Manipulation, Definitive Physiotherapy excluding manipulation, Corset and Analgesics. Patients received a minimum of two treatments per week for three weeks unless complete relief was attained. The patient's assessments of pain after three weeks of treatment are shown in Table VI-1. Doran and Newell analyzed these data using the chi-square test and found no significant effects. However, the chi-square test is not appropriate for this sort of data because it views the assessments of pain as six unrelated categories rather than as a six-point ordinal scale ranging from "worse" to "completely relieved." Greenland et al (1980) have noted that when more appropriate statistical tests are used (e.g. the Mann-Whitney U test and the Kruskal-Wallis analysis of variance), the results tend to favor spinal manipulation as a treatment for low back pain. Furthermore, there appeared to be a small number of patients who greatly benefitted from manipulation. Forty of the 68 patients who dropped out of the study were in the manipulated group. Twenty-six of these said that they stopped treatment because they felt better. There were no apparent prognostic features distinguishing these patients from the rest of the population (Doran and Newell, 1975; Newell, 1977).

It should be noted that this study has been severely criticized on the grounds that (1) the investigators did not properly select patients who

Table VI-1

PATIENT'S ASSESSMENTS OF PAIN AT THREE WEEKS

	Manipulation	Physiotherapy	Corset	Analgesics
Worse	6	9	5	7
Unchanged	12	21	24	24
Slightly improved	17	20	18	20
Moderately improved	19	18	19	13
Markedly improved	30	26	24	23
Completely relieved	14	10	3	13
Total	98	104	93	100

From Doran and Newell (1975)

would be most suitable for manipulation therapy (Boag, 1975; Cyriax, 1975; Riches, 1975) and (2) the clinicians did not have sufficient training in spinal manipulation (Ebbets, 1975).

Bergquist-Ullman and Larsson

A study on low back pain in industry, conducted by Bergquist-Ullman and Larsson (1977), included an evaluation of manipulative treatment versus a "back school" or placebo diathermy. Unfortunately the "manipulated" group actually received various types of physiotherapy including exercises, mobilization and various types of manipulative therapy and therefore does not provide a clear indication of the effect of manipulation. Patients in the combined physiotherapy group had a mean duration of symptoms of 15.8 days as compared to 14.8 days in the "back school" group and 28.7 days in the placebo group. Statistical analyses indicated that the placebo group was significantly worse than the other two treatment methods. No significant differences were observed in any other measures of the effect of treatment.

Evans et al

A clinical trial reported by Evans et al (1978) and Roberts et al (1978) employed a crossover design in which 32 low-back pain patients were studied for a total of 42 days. One group of patients (Group A) received rotational manipulation of the lumbar spine on Days 0, 7 and 14 while the other group (Group B) received manipulative therapy on Days 21, 28 and 35. Patients were allowed analgesics (codeine) throughout the entire study and therefore this clinical trial represents a comparison between manipulation plus analgesics and analgesics alone. Manipulative treatment was described as "a rotational thrust with distraction both to the right and to the left." The results of this study are shown in Table VI-2 which presents the mean subjective pain scores reported during the various conditions and Table VI-3 which presents a measurement of anterior spinal flexion using the method of Macrae and Wright (1967). Manipulation apparently produced a decrease in subjective pain and an increase in the capacity for anterior spinal flexion. Unfortunately, the statistical significance of these results is unclear. Crossover designs are always problematic because of the possibility that a carryover effect of the first treatment received will obfuscate comparisons involving the second treatment. For example, if manipulation were to produce a permanent cure for back pain, patients who were cured by the initial

Table VI-2

TOTAL PAIN SCORES OF EACH GROUP DIVIDED
BY THE NUMBER OF PATIENTS IN THE GROUP

Group	Total pain scores in					
	week 1	week 2	week 3	week 4	week 5	week 6
A	Manipulation			Control		
	12.20	10.87	10.47	10.00	10.93	10.40
B	Control			Manipulation		
	9.59	8.88	9.53	9.35	8.53	8.71

From Evans et al (1978)

Table VI-3

ANTERIOR SPINAL FLEXION MEASUREMENTS
(USING METHOD OF MACRAE AND WRIGHT, 1969)

Group	Median (range) anterior spinal flexion (cm)		
	Baseline	Day 21	Day 42
A	5.2(2.6-7.1)	5.4(3.5-8.9)	5.2(3.8-6.6)
B	6.1(3.0-9.1)	5.8(2.0-9.0)	6.3(2.6-9.8)

From Evans et al (1978)

manipulative treatment would also appear to be "cured" after a subsequent placebo treatment. Such a phenomenon may, in fact, have occured in Group A. These difficulties are exacerbated if, as is the case in the Evans et al (1978) trial, there are baseline differences between the two groups.

The most obvious statistical test of the efficacy of manipulation is a paired comparison involving all patients, in which scores obtained following manipulation are compared with scores obtained following control treatment. Thus, each patient serves as his own control. These analyses were not reported and we can only assume that they were not statistically significant. In and of itself, this would not indicate that manipulation was no different from control. Because of the apparent carryover effect in Group A, the statistical significance of the difference between groups will tend to be underestimated. A proper analysis would require a paired comparison using analysis of covariance to adjust for baseline levels of pain and anterior flexion.

Overall, 14 patients reported themselves to be "markedly improved" while 7 were "slightly improved," 6 were unchanged and 2 were worse. By comparing the 14 "markedly improved" patients (responders) with the 8 who were unchanged or worse (non-responders), Evans et al (1978) attempted to assess the role of various prognostic factors in predicting the response to manipulation. Responders tended to be older (median age: 50 vs. 36.5 years) with a shorter duration of back pain (median: 3 vs. 10 years) and a later age at onset (median: 43.1 vs. 26.5 years).

Rasmussen

Rasmussen (1979) reported a clinical trial in which 24 patients with back pain of less than 3 weeks duration were randomly assigned to receive either rotational manipulation in the pain-free direction or shortwave diathermy. All patients received 3 treatments per week for 2 weeks. At the end of the 14-day treatment period, 11 of 12 manipulation patients but only 3 of 12 control patients reported complete cessation of symptoms. All 12 manipulated patients but only 6 of 12 control patients showed improvement in a modified Schober's test, similar to the anterior flexion test used by Evans et al (1978). Both of these effects were highly significant ($p < .01$). The better results obtained in this study can probably be attributed to the exclusion of chronic back-pain patients who appear to be less likely to respond to manipulation.

Jayson et al

Mobilization and manipulation using the techniques of Maitland (1977) were studied in a clinical trial reported by Jayson et al (1981) and Sims-Williams et al (1978; 1979). A total of 188 patients were admitted to the study; 94 were referred from general practitioners and 94 were referred from hospital clinics. Patients were randomly assigned to receive either mobilization and manipulation or simulated diathermy. Assessments were performed at the end of the one month course of treatment and at 3 and 12 months. Variables assessed included subjective pain, physical activity, the patient's opinions of treatment, anterior and lateral flexion, extension and straight leg raising. The measures of spinal mobility utilized the methods of Loebl (1967) and Reynolds (1975). At the end of treatment, the general practitioner patients appeared to obtain somewhat greater clinical benefits from mobilization/manipulation than from simulated diathermy but this effect was not statistically significant. There was little effect of manipulative treatment on hospital patients. Both the general practitioner patients and the hospital patients showed significant increases in the angle of straight leg raising after mobilization/manipulation while the control treatment had no effect. However, the 3- and 12-month assessments did not reveal any differences between manipulated and control patients.

As in previous clinical trials of manipulation, Jayson et al (1981) searched for prognostic variables that might predict the response to treatment. The only variable of any importance was the duration of pain. Patients with a long history of pain were less likely to benefit from manipulation.

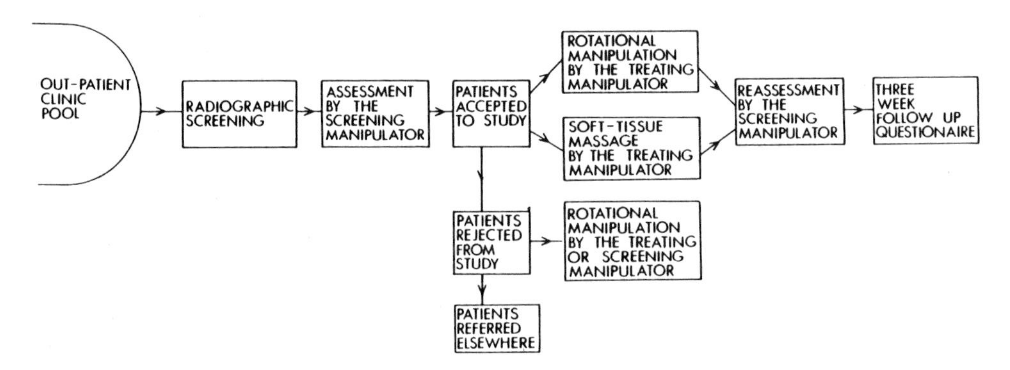

Figure VI-3. The design of the University of California, Irvine, clinical trial of spinal manipulation for low-back pain.

Hoehler et al

The first controlled trial of spinal manipulation to be conducted in the United States was reported by Buerger (1980) and Hoehler, Tobis and Buerger (1981). This study is particularly noteworthy because it was the first clinical trial of manipulation to use an appropriate placebo treatment on the control group. The experimental group received rotational manipulations of the lumbosacral spine while the control group received soft-tissue massage of the same area. In order to assure the validity of this placebo treatment, patients who had previous experience with manipulative therapy were excluded from the study. The design of this study is shown in Figure VI-3. Figure VI-4 shows the proportion of patients claiming relief of pain and improvement in the ability to perform various activities requiring spinal flexibility. These effects were seen immediately after the first treatment.

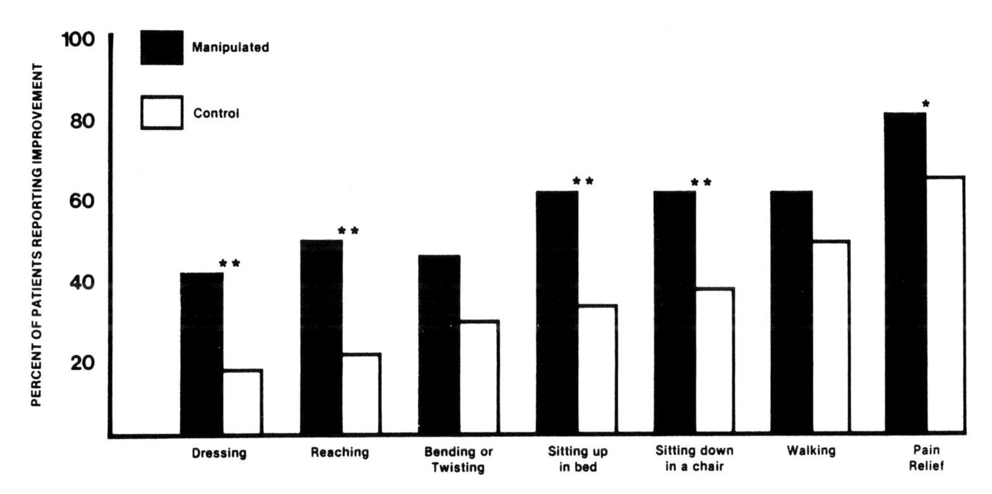

Figure VI-4. Percentage of patients reporting improvement on various measures of spinal flexibility immediately after manipulative therapy on soft-tissue massage (control) ** = $p < .01$, * = $p < .05$ (from Tobis and Hoehler, 1983).

By the time of discharge from the clinic, there was no difference between groups because both had shown substantial improvement: 88% of the manipulated patients and 86% of the controls claimed that their treatment had been effective. However, 3 weeks after discharge, manipulated patients were significantly more likely than controls to report that the treatment had been effective. Figure VI-5 shows improvements in the straight leg raising test both immediately after the first manipulative treatment and at the time of discharge fom the clinic. Again, manipulation produced significantly more improvement than the control treatment, immediately after the first treatment. However, at discharge, there was no difference between the two groups because both were greatly improved.

This clinical trial was the first to provide evidence of the validity of the control procedure. Three weeks after discharge, patients were asked whether they thought they had received spinal manipulation or soft tissue massage. There was no difference between the groups: 66% of the manipulated patients thought they had received spinal manipulation while 56% of the control patients thought that they had received spinal manipulation. Thus, in this trial, the soft-tissue-massage control treatment appeared to function as an adequate placebo for manipulative therapy.

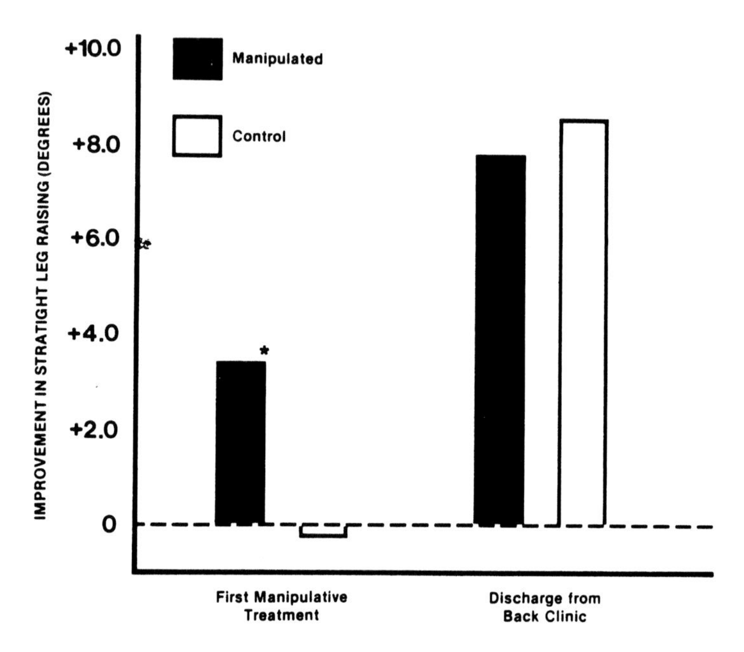

Figure VI-5. Effect of manipulative therapy vs soft-tissue massage (control) on increases in the angle of straight-leg raising immediately after the initial treatment and at the time of discharge from the back clinic. * = $p < .05$ (from Tobis and Hoehler, 1983).

Coxhead

Coxhead et al (1981) conducted a multicenter study on various types of physiotherapy in patients with sciatica with or without low back pain. Physiotherapeutic methods used included Exercises, Traction, Corset and Manipulation using the methods of Maitland (1977). Outpatients at eight hospitals in and around London were randomly assigned to one of 16 groups that received every possible combination of 0, 1, 2, 3 or all of these 4 treatments. All patients received short-wave diathermy as placebo. In order to examine the effects of manipulation, manipulated

Table VI-4

PATIENT'S ASSESSMENTS AT FOUR WEEKS BY TYPE OF TREATMENT

		Traction		Manipulation		Exercises		Corset	
	–	Yes	No	Yes	No	Yes	No	Yes	No
Better	No.	117	110	127	100	120	107	100	127
	%	82	74	82	73	80	75	81	76
Same	No.	19	28	18	29	19	28	16	31
	%	13	19	12	21	13	20	13	18
Worse	No.	7	11	10	8	11	7	8	10
	%	5	7	6	6	7	5	6	6
Total	No.	143	149	155	137	150	142	124	168
	%	100	100	100	100	100	100	100	100

From Coxhead et al (1981)

Table VI-5

MEAN IMPROVEMENT (±SD) AT FOUR WEEKS
ON -100 TO +100 SCALE BY TREATMENT

Traction		Manipulation		Exercises		Corset	
Yes	No	Yes	No	Yes	No	Yes	No
50.1	45.4	52.6	42.2	49.0	46.3	49.8	46.1
(37.9)	(40.3)	(36.9)	(40.9)	(40.0)	(38.2)	(37.9)	(40.0)

From Coxhead et al (1981)

patients were compared to patients who did not receive manipulation. Both of these groups contained many patients who had received one or more of the other therapeutic procedures. Data on patient improvement at 4 months are shown in Table VI-6. Although Coxhead et al reported no significant differences, a re-analysis using the Mann-Whitney U test with correction for ties indicates a marginally significant beneficial effect of manipulation as compared to control at 4 weeks ($p = .044$). The mean extent of relief at 4 weeks is shown in Table VI-5. Manipulation was significantly better than control ($p < .05$). It is unfortunate that Coxhead et

Table VI-6

PATIENT'S ASSESSMENTS AT FOUR MONTHS BY TYPE OF TREATMENT

		Traction		Manipulation		Exercises		Corset	
	–	Yes	No	Yes	No	Yes	No	Yes	No
Better	No.	89	92	100	81	85	96	78	103
	%	72	72	75	70	69	76	71	74
Same	No.	27	24	22	29	29	22	23	28
	%	22	19	16	25	23	17	21	20
Worse	No.	7	11	12	6	10	8	9	9
	%	6	9	9	5	8	6	8	6
Total	No.	123	127	134	116	124	126	110	140
	%	100	100	100	100	100	100	100	100

From Coxhead et al (1981)

al did not report the results of each of the 16 treatment combinations. A proper statistical analysis (2×2×2×2 factorial analysis of variance) would have allowed an assessment of the main effects of each individual treatment as well as the effects of any interaction between treatments. Because Coxhead et al (1981) reported that the extent of improvement was a direct function of the number of different treatments employed, we may surmise that there were some significant interactions. However, the nature of these effects is unclear.

Sloop et al

Sloop et al (1982) reported a clinical trial that is most notable for its unusual approach to the problem of the development of a valid control procedure for studies of spinal manipulation. Patients were given an amnesic dose of i.v. diazepam in order to prevent them from remembering whether they had received manipulation therapy. This is also, to our knowledge, the only clinical trial of cervical rather than lumbar manipulation for spinal pain although there are several clinical trials of cervical manipulation as a treatment for migraine (Parker et al 1978) and other pathological conditions. Unfortunately, the number of patients employed in this study was too small to produce reliable results. Twelve of 21 manipulated patients (57%) claimed that the treatment had helped them while only 5 of 18 untreated patients (28%) reported beneficial effects. This is a substantial difference between groups but, given the low numbers of patients, it was not sufficient to yield statistical significance. An additional problem is that results obtained on manipulation performed in conjunction with i.v. diazepam might not be particularly relevant to the typical clinical situation in which manipulation is usually performed without such pharmaceutical intervention. Thus, despite its interesting methodology, this study is not particularly informative regarding the efficacy of spinal manipulation.

Nwuga

In a clinical trial conducted in Nigeria, Nwuga (1982) investigated spinal manipulation in the treatment of female patients with acute low back pain (duration < 2 weeks) believed to result from rupture of the intervertebral disc. The entrance criteria are noteworthy because, although Cyriax (1971) recommends manipulation as a treatment for herniated disc, most of the studies previously described (Glover et al, 1974; Doran and Newell, 1975; Evans et al, 1978; Rasmussen, 1979; Jayson et al, 1981; Hoehler et al, 1981) have excluded patients with apparent disc involvement.

Nwuga (1982) employed a manipulative technique described as "lumbar oscillatory rotation" (Nwuga, 1976) which was "effected by the therapist's hand nudging the upper half of the buttocks in a push-relax sequence to the point of pain." Control patients received shortwave diathermy followed by isometric exercises. All patients received instruction in posture and the mechanics of lifting. Treatments were given three times a week until pain was no longer present. A total of 51 patients (26 manipulated and 25 controls) were treated in this clinical trial.

Six weeks after the start of treatment, all patients were assessed by a clinician who did not know which treatment the patient had received. The results indicated a substantial therapeutic effect of manipulation on range of motion (Table VI-7) and straight-leg raising (Table VI-8). The highly significant improvements observed in this study indicate that either (1) Nwuga's methods of manipulation are superior to those previously investigated or (2) patients with a clinically diagnosed herniated disc are more likely to improve as a result of spinal manipulation therapy. It should be noted that Nwuga's patients had considerable room for improvement. For example, the mean angle of straight leg raising was 29° prior to treatment and 68° after manipulative therapy. In the clinical trial reported by Hoehler, Tobis, and Buerger (1981) initial straight leg raising angles were much higher (64°) and the amount of improvement was correspondingly less.

Table VI-7

MEAN AND STANDARD ERROR OF THE MEAN (±) OF
PRE-TREATMENT AND POST-TREATMENT RANGE OF MOTION

Motion	Group	Pre-Treatment mean	Post-Treatment mean	p-value
Total flexion and	Control	32° ± 1.5	45° ± 1.9	0.10
extension	Manipulated	33° ± 1.9	67° ± 2.1	0.005
Total side flexion	Control	35° ± 1.4	38° ± 2.1	NS
	Manipulated	37° ± 1.8	46° ± 1.7	0.05
Total rotation	Control	8° ± 2.1	10° ± 2.2	NS
	Manipulated	9° ± 1.5	16° ± 1.3	0.05

NS = Not Significant

From Nwuga (1982)

Table VI-8

STRAIGHT-LEG RAISING VALUES
PRE-TREATMENT AND POST-TREATMENT

Group	Pre-treatment	Post-treatment	p-value
Control	31° ± 1.8	35° ± 2.3	NS
Manipulated	29° ± 2.1	68° ± 1.9	0.01

NS = Not Significant

From Nwuga (1982)

Farrell and Twomey

In an Australian clinical trial reported by Farrell and Twomey (1982) 24 low back pain patients received three manipulative treatments per week for up to three weeks while 24 patients received a control treatment consisting of short-wave diathermy, isometric abdominal exercises and ergonomic instruction. The experimental treatment was described as "passive mobilization and manipulation" using the techniques described by Stoddard (1979) and Maitland (1977).

The manipulated patients required a mean of 3.5 treatments to reach a symptom-free status while the control group required 5.8 treatments for remission of symptoms. This difference was statistically significant. The manipulated group also displayed a significantly greater capacity for lumbar extension. Multivariate analyses indicated that the most reliable predictor of the success of treatment was duration of back pain.

Godfrey et al

Godfrey et al (1984) recently conducted a randomized controlled clinical trial of manipulation using the methods of Maigne (1972) both for the methods of treatment and the assessment of its effects. A total of 81 patients participated in the study. A major entry criterion was a "restriction of motion in two or more noncontiguous planes" as described by Maigne (1972) and the major response variable was elimination or reduction of that restriction. The course of manipulative therapy was agreed upon by a physician and a chiropractor and was briefly described as "a brisk rotational thrust in the direction away from the greatest restriction." Upon entry into the study, patients were randomized to one of four groups; (a) manipulation and soft-tissue massage alone (N=22), (b) manipulation and placebo electrostimulation (N=22), (c) massage alone (N=20), or (d) electrostimulation alone (N=17). After a maximum of five treatments, the patient was re-examined by an assessor who was not aware of the nature of the treatments employed.

Unfortunately, this apparently well-controlled trial was not analyzed properly. Like several previous studies (Doran & Newell, 1975; Jayson et al, 1981), the authors used chi-square tests on ordinal scales of patient improvement. As noted by Greenland et al (1980), simple chi-square tests are not appropriate in such cases because they ignore all information regarding the order of the quantitative scale. Thus, although the authors report no significant effects of manipulation, re-analysis to the extent possible from the published data, using an appropriate statistical test (the Mann-Whitney U Test with a correction for ties) indicated that manipulation produced significant ($p < .05$) improvement in range of motion. In the manipulated group 29% of the patients showed marked improvement while 80% showed at least moderate improvement on that measure. In contrast, only 14% of control patients showed marked improvement and 60% showed at least moderate improvement. Thus, despite the author's conclusions, this study provides further evidence for the efficiency of spinal manipulation.

Summary

Table VI-9 summarizes the fourteen clinical trials of spinal manipulation that we have discussed above. In order to present a consistent measure of clinical efficacy, the percentage of patients improved was determined by us using published data where available. Fisher's exact test for 2 by 2 tables was used for statistical analysis. It is apparent that these studies are characterized by a wide variety of patient populations, methods of treatment and methods of response assessment. However, there is, clearly, a general tendency for patients to improve more rapidly following manipulative therapy. A recent review of conservative therapy for low-back pain agreed with this assessment but noted that none of the clinical trials of any conservative therapeutic modality meets rigorous criteria for validity and applicability (Deyo, 1983). Even with relaxed standards, only two of these studies (Hoehler et al, 1981; Farrell and Twomey, 1982) were considered to be adequate. In order for clinical trials of spinal manipulation to be truly acceptable, more attention must be paid to blinding of patients and examiners and standardization of patient entry criteria, therapeutic methodology, and outcome measurement.

An additional clinical trial of spinal manipulation has come to our attention.[1] In this study, conducted at Guy's Hospital, London, manipulative treatment by "a nonmedical qualified osteopath" was compared to short-wave diathermy and placebo diathermy administered by a phsiotherapist. A total of 109 hospital outpatients with nonspecific low back pain of 2-12 months duration participated in the study. Osteopathic treatment "included examination, soft-tissue manipulation, passive articulation of stiff spinal segments, and manipulation of the vertebral facet of sacroiliac joints using minimal rotation." Indices of

1. Gibson T, Grahame R, Harkness J, Woo P, Blagrave P, and Hills R. Controlled comparison of short-wave diathermy treatment with osteopathic treatment in nonspecific low back pain. *Lancet*, 1:1258-1261, 1985.

pain and range of motion were not significantly different in the three treatment groups. However, it should be noted that this study constitutes a clinical trial of the manipulative techniques of only one osteopath and, therefore, its general applicability may be questioned.

Table VI-9

CLINICAL TRIALS OF MANIPULATION

STUDY	PATIENTS	MANIPULATION	CONTROL	TIME	NUMBER OF PATIENTS MAN.	NUMBER OF PATIENTS CON.	PERCENT IMPROVED MAN.	PERCENT IMPROVED CON.	*p*
Coyer & Curwen 1955	Patients presenting to St Thomas's Hospital, London with recent low-back pain.	Methods of Cyriax	Analgesia and bedrest	1 wk 3 wks 6 wks	76 76 76	60 60 60	50 87 88	27 60 72	.005 <.001 <.014
Glover et al 1974	Employees of the Westinghouse Brake and Signal Co. Ltd, Chippenham Wiltshire reporting to the works medical center with unilateral low back pain.	Rotational manipulation of the lower spine.	Detuned Diathermy	immed-1 wk	43	41	--	--	--*
Doran & Newell 1975	Patients with back pain reporting to Departments of Rheumatology at 7 hospitals in Britain and Wales.	At the discretion of the manipulator.	Physiotherapy corset or analgesics	3 wks 6 wks 3 mths	98 92 93	297 244 242	64 65 74	50 67 74	.010 NS NS
Bergquist-Ullman & Larsson, 1977	Employees of AB Volvo, Goteborg, Sweden with acute or subacute low-back pain of less than three months duration.	Mobilization, exercises or manipulation using various methods.	"Back School" or microwave diathermy.	0–6 wks	68	129	--	--	--**
Evans et al 1978	Patients presenting to the University Hospital of Wales, Cardiff with low back pain persisting for at least 3 weeks.	Rotational thrust with distraction both to the right and to the left.	Analgesics	3 wks	15	17	60	18	.017
Jayson et al 1978	Patients with low back pain seen by various British general practioners.	Methods of Maitland	Microwave Radiation	1 mth 3 mths	43 40	44 43	91 65	73 51	.028 NS

Table VI-9 *(Continued)*

STUDY	PATIENTS	MANIPULATION	CONTROL	TIME	NUMBER OF PATIENTS		PERCENT IMPROVED		*p*
					MAN.	CON.	MAN.	CON.	
Jayson et al 1979	Patients with low back pain referred to various British hospital rheumatologic or orthopedic clinics.	Methods of Maitland	Microwave Radiation	1 mth	47	43	62	58	NS
				3 mths	42	40	67	68	NS
Rasmussen 1979	Patients presenting to the department of Physical Medicine and Rheumatology, Aalborg Hospital, Denmark, with back pain persisting for less than 3 weeks.	Rotational manipulation in the pain-free direction.	Short wave diathermy	1 wk	12	12	58	17	.045
				3 wks	12	12	92	25	.001
Hoehler et al 1981	Patients referred to the University of California, Irvine Medical Center, Back Clinic with low back pain.	Rotational Manipulation, Methods of Fisk	Soft-tissue massage	Immed	56	38	84	68	.065
				Approx. 3 wks	41	28	83	71	NS
				Approx. 3 mths	33	25	79	52	.031
Coxhead et al 1981	Patients presenting to one of 8 hospitals in and around London with pain of sciatic distribution with or without back pain.	Methods of Maitland	Traction, exercises, corset or microwave diathermy	4 wks	155	137	82	73	.046
				4 mths	134	116	75	70	NS
Sloop et al 1982	Patients referred to Northwick Park Hospital, Middlesex, England with neck pain.	Cervical Manipulation Using Methods of Cyriax, Maigne, Maitland under i.v. diazepam.	i.v. diazepam only	3 wks	21	18	57	28	.064

Table VI-9 *(Continued)*

STUDY	PATIENTS	MANIPULATION	CONTROL	TIME	NUMBER OF PATIENTS MAN.	NUMBER OF PATIENTS CON.	PERCENT IMPROVED MAN.	PERCENT IMPROVED CON.	*p*
Nwuga 1982	Female patients referred to the Physical Therapy Department, Ife University Teaching Hospitals Complex, Ile-Ife, Nigeria with back pain and sciatica resulting from a ruptured intervertebral disc.	Lumbar oscillating rotation as described by Nwuga.	Short-wave diathermy	4 wks	26	25	--	--	--***
Farrell et al 1982	Patients presenting to School of Physiotherapy, Western Australia Institute of Technology with low back pain of less than 3 weeks duration.	Methods of Stoddard and Maitland	Microwave diathermy	1 wk	24	24	17	8	NS
				2 wks	24	24	67	29	.001
				3 wks	24	24	92	63	.030
				4 wks	24	24	96	88	NS
Godfrey et al 1984	Patients with acute non-specific back pain and restricted motion referred to the Department of Rehabilitation Medicine, Wellesley Hospital, Toronto.	Methods of Maigne	Massage and electrostimulation	2 wks	41	35	80	60	.044

p values were determined by us using Fisher's exact test for 2 by 2 Tables (one-sided). NS = not significant

* In a subgroup of patients with acute low back pain, manipulation produced significantly ($p < .05$) more relief than control immediately after treatment but not at 3 or 7 days.

** Mean duration of symptoms were: Manipulation: 15.8 days; Back School: 14.8 days; Placebo: 28.7 days.

*** Manipulation produced significantly greater increases in straight-leg raising ($p < .01$), side-flexion ($p < .05$) and rotation ($p < .05$) than control.

CHAPTER VII

HOW DOES MANIPULATION WORK?

THE CLINICAL TRIAL data presented in the preceding chapter clearly indicate that spinal manipulation works. That is, manipulated patients are significantly more likely to improve than those patients receiving one of several different types of control management. The obvious question, then, is how does it work? Unfortunately, research has not yet provided any definite, or even suggestive, evidence pointing toward the answer to this question. It is safe to say that the correction of each of the possible causes of back pain discussed in Chapter II has been suggested as a candidate for the mechanism of action of manipulation. However, scientific evidence is scarce. This is not surprising considering the orientation towards clinical practice rather than research that has generally characterized the osteopathic and chiropractic professions which are most closely identified with spinal manipulation. The competition between these professions and organized medicine has insured that the large research-oriented hospitals and medical schools in the United States remain hostile to studies on manipulative medicine (Wardwell, 1972). In fact, at this date, our 1981 study, remains the first and only published controlled clinical trial of spinal manipulation conducted in the United States.

The neglect of research on spinal manipulation certainly cannot be attributed to the absence of international, interdisciplinary conferences on the subject. The first major meeting, entitled "The Research Status of Spinal Manipulative Therapy," was held under the auspices of the National Institute of Neurological and Communicative Disorders and Stroke of the National Institute of Health in 1975 (Goldstein, 1975). Later in that same year, an institutional conference on Approaches to the Validation of Manipulation Therapy was held at the University of California, Irvine, California (Buerger and Tobis, 1977). In 1977, Michigan

State University—the only university in the United States offering both the M.D. and the D.O. degrees on one campus held its first workshop on the Research Status of Spinal Manipulative Therapy (Korr, 1978). The most recent such meeting at Michigan State University was held in 1983 (Gunby, 1983). However, there is still very little solid evidence regarding the reasons for the efficacy of spinal manipulation. Below, we discuss some of the data in support of various putative mechanisms of back pain that may be relieved by manipulation.

Nerve Compression

The early chiropractic notion that vertebral subluxations produced pathological effects through simple nerve compression and that manipulation relieved this compression by adjusting the vertebrae has been generally discredited. For example, Crelin's (1973) study showed that, in cadavers, subluxations sufficient to embarrass the intervertebral foramen could not be made to occur. However, this is one of the most naive and ancient of chiropractic theories and its disproof has little relevance for the more complex and sophisticated models of vertebral subluxations.

One anatomically more likely means of nerve compression involves spasm of the piriformis muscle which crosses over and, in some cases, surrounds the sciatic nerve (Pace and Nagle, 1976; Retzloff et al, 1974). In a pilot study of the effects of manipulation on spinal reflexes, we studied two patients with piriformis syndrome who were treated by rectal digital massage of the affected muscle. These patients, whose reflexes were absent on the affected side, showed no change after treatment (Hoehler, 1981).

Disc Involvement

It has been suggested that the intervertebral disc is responsible for most cases of nonspecific low back pain (Nachemson, 1976). As we have previously noted, Cyriax (1971, 1982) has always claimed that the beneficial effects of spinal manipulation result from the repositioning of displaced fragments of an intervertebral disc.

Coyer and Curwen (1955) have concluded that the basis for the efficacy of manipulation is the result of action on the disc. They have stated that, "In the patient with acute low back pain in whom the probable lesion is derangement of an intervertebral joint, including minor protrusion of a disk, and in whom irritation or pressure on adjacent structures occurs, then treatment by manipulation, without anaesthesia seems a logical method of gaining relief from signs and symptoms." However, there is little direct evidence for this proposition. Studies have shown both increases (Wilson and Ilfeld, 1952) and decreases (Mathews and Yates, 1969) in the size of myelographic deficits following spinal manipulation. Furthermore, in the group studied by Chrisman et al (1964), patients with no demonstrable myelographic defect showed the best response to manipulative treatment. Thus, there is no convincing evidence that manipulation operates through action on the intervertebral disc.

Mechanical Derangements of the Spine

It has often been suggested that the effects of spinal manipulation result from the correction of minor mechanical derangements of the spinal column. The structures responsible for pain are generally believed to be either the facet joints or the ligaments. Glover (1960) reported that back pain was often characterized by a localized hyperesthesia which he attributed to facet joint impaction. When the patient was successfully treated by spinal manipulation, both the back pain and the hyperesthesia were eliminated. However, objective evidence via radiography has not been obtained. Roberts et al (1978) found no radiographic changes following spinal manipulation while Hoehler and Tobis (1982), found no effects of manipulation on posture as measured by iliac and scapular levels. It should be noted however that radiographic techniques are limited and are unlikely to detect minor alterations in the spinal column (Swezey and Silverman, 1971). More sensitive measures such as magnetic resonance imaging may be indicated here but, as yet there is little evidence that manipulation affects the mechanical relationships of the spinal column.

Reflex Muscle Spasm

One of the most popular theories of manipulation is based on the hypothesis that most low-back pain results from muscle spasm. Because the pain also causes continued muscle spasm, a "vicious circle" is initiated. Manipulation presumably interrupts this process by stretching the muscles and eliminating spasm. Buerger (1983) has noted that tetanization of isolated muscle preparations results in a long-acting potentiation of stretch receptor discharge. This discharge—which could, in an intact organism, produce muscle spasm—is reduced by stretching the muscle.

This is a plausible model for the effects of manipulation on back pain but there is no direct evidence connecting clinical experience to the experimental model. A more complex and realistic model of back pain may be the artificially induced muscle soreness that can result from rigorous muscular activity. De Vries (1961, 1966) found that static stretch of muscle reduced both electromyographic activity and subjective pain. However, McGlynn (1975) reported that, although EMG activity was reduced following static stretch, subjective pain was no different than that reported by the control group.

Psychological Factors

Many who provide clinical care to patients with low-back pain express skepticism about the efficacy of manipulation as having a true physiological effect. Thus there is a widespread belief that the "green poultice" in workmen's compensation can result in dramatic improvement in the patient's complaints.

To date, no well-controlled study has addressed the importance of the psychological variables in determining the therapeutic efficacy of manipulation. However, psychological differences in patients with back pain have been well documented and numerous psychological models of back pain have been proposed (Turk and Flor, 1984). In the next chapter we address this matter in greater detail, reporting on a study we conducted concerning neurotic behavior patterns related to the treatment of back pain by spinal manipulation.

CHAPTER VIII

WHO CAN BENEFIT FROM MANIPULATION?

IT IS APPARENT that, like most medical treatments, spinal manipulation is not universally effective. Unfortunately, there has been little success in predicting the outcome of manipulative therapy in individual patients. Indeed, Fisk (1977) has suggested that, with the exception of patients for whom manipulation is contraindicated for reasons of safety, all individuals with low back pain should be treated by manipulation. Thus, the applicability of treatment is determined by simply performing the treatment.

Clinical trials of manipulation have not been particularly helpful. Doran and Newell (1975) stated that there was no relationship between the physician's initial assessment and the extent of pain relief produced by manipulation, or any other treatment. Buerger (1980) reported a statistically significant correlation between the physician's initial assessment of manipulability and the patient's eventual response to manipulation. However, the magnitude of the correlation coefficient was rather low (r_s = .137). Thus, it appears that clinicians can distinguish those patients who are likely to do well although the rate of error is high and the basis for the distinction is not well understood.

Diagnostic Features of Back Pain—Disc Involvement

Most clinical trials of spinal manipulation appear to have excluded patients with signs of a possible herniated disc (Glover et al, 1974; Doran & Newell, 1975; Evans et al, 1978; Rasmussen, 1979; Jayson et al, 1981; Hoehler et al, 1981; Farrell and Twomey, 1982). However, it is interesting to note that the two studies which did admit such patients were those that yielded the most impressive effects of spinal manipulation. Coyer and Curwen (1955) reported that approximately half of their patients had restricted straight-leg raising which they considered to indicate the presence of a disk lesion. Nwuga (1982) admitted only patients with a definitive diagnosis of herniated nucleus pulposus and reported substantial improvements in measures of flexability as compared to the far more modest improvements reported in other studies (Doran & Newell, 1975; Evans et al, 1978; Jayson et al, 1981; Hoehler et al, 1981; Farrell and Twomey, 1982). This suggests that the effects of manipulation in cases with disk involvement should be further investigated.

Duration of Back Pain

One factor which has consistently been correlated with the efficacy of spinal manipulation is the duration of back pain prior to treatment. Most studies which have had a wide range of pain durations have reported that patients with shorter durations of treatment tend to be more responsive to manipulation (Glover et al, 1974; Evans et al, 1978; Jayson et al, 1981; Hoehler and Tobis, 1983; Farrell and Twomey, 1982). In one study, shorter durations of pain did not predict the ultimate level of pain relief but did predict a shorter total duration of treatment (Hoehler et al, 1981).

Demographic and Other Variables

In one study (Evans et al, 1978) it was reported that patients who were older, and had a greater age at onset of back pain, were more likely to respond to manipulative treatment. No other study has reported age to be a significant prognostic variable. The exact nature of all variables shown to be unrelated to the effects of spinal manipulation can not be exactly determined from published reports. Many reports simply state that a large number of variables were examined and found to be unrelated (Doran & Newell, 1975; Jayson et al, 1981; Hoehler et al, 1981). We may presume, however, that these include age, sex and pretreatment measures of flexibility.

Psychological Factors

As noted in the previous chapter, back pain is a disorder that is generally believed to have important psychological components. The characteristics of "psychosomatic" back pain are not well understood and explanations include conscious or unconscious "malingering" for secondary gain (Finneson, 1976), stress-induced "tension myositis" (Sarno,

1981), and a "pain-fear" syndrome resulting in extreme immobilization which prevents recovery (Caldwell and Chase, 1977). One promising avenue for research on psychological factors in back pain involves the use of standardized measures of personality on back-pain patients. In an early study using the Minnesota Multiphasic Personality Inventory (MMPI), Hanvik (1951) compared a group of patients with organic back pain to a group of patients with functional back pain and noted the appearance of a configuration typical of conversion hysteria in the functional patients. This configuration is characterized by high scores on Hypochondriasis and Hysteria and relatively lower scores on Depression. In general, functional back pain has been shown to be reliably correlated with neuroticism as measured by the MMPI, although the results obtained from other personality inventories have been somewhat less consistent (Crown, 1978).

Elevated indices of neuroticism appear to be correlated with a relatively poor response to medical or surgical treatments for back pain. High scores on the Hs and Hy scales of the MMPI have been shown to indicate an unfavorable prognosis for spinal fusion (Wilfing et al, 1973), chemonucleolysis (Wiltse, and Rocchio, 1975), neurosurgical treatment (Blumetti and Modesti, 1976) and "conservative" treatment (McCreary et al, 1979). It has also been shown that high scores on the somatic, obsessional and depressive scales of the Middlesex Hospital Questionnaire (MHQ) tend to predict a poor response to physical therapy (Wolkind and Forrest, 1972), although another study indicated that the MHQ failed to identify those back pain patients who became persistent attendees at a rheumatology clinic (Lloyd et al, 1979).

We have used a short form of the MMPI in an attempt to predict the response to spinal manipulation. The extent of relief from back pain was assessed immediately after manipulative treatment and, again, approximately five days later. It has often been noted that some patients may report immediate relief from pain only to have the pain return within days or even hours of an apparently successful spinal manipulation (Fisk, 1977). Two hypotheses present themselves. First, it is possible that the immediate relief is psychologically produced and, therefore, tends to dissipate when the patient is removed from the presence of the clinician. Alternatively, manipulation may break the "pain-fear" cycle but, in the neurotic patient, this may be only temporary. If the former it would be highly correlated with the amount of immediate relief reported. In contrast, the latter hypothesis predicts that psychological factors will only be correlated with the extent of the more permanent relief from pain.

In our investigations of the effect of psychological factors in low back pain (Hoehler & Tobis, 1983) we examined a sample of 90 patients who were treated by spinal manipulation in the Back Clinic of the University of California Irvine Medical Center between 1975 and 1979. These patients were diagnosed by the examining physician as having non-specific low back pain with a restricted range of motion that might be amenable to manipulative therapy.

The therapy employed here involved rotational manipulation of the lumbosacral spine as described in Chapter VI (Fisk, 1977).

The psychological inventory consisted of Kincannon's (1968) 71-item Mini-Mult with the addition of 17 items required to complete Hanvik's (1951) functional low back pain scale. Although the Mini-Mult is not adequate clinical replacement for the MMPI, the correlations between MMPI and Mini-Mult scores are quite high, and the test would seem to be valid for a comparison of groups (Tsushima, 1975).

All Mini-Mult scores were converted to MMPI equivalents and then to standard scores. A score of 50 is generally considered to be "normal," while a score of 70 or greater is believed to indicate substantial pathology. Two measures of "improvement" were used. Immediately after the first treatment, patients were asked:

> How does your present pain or discomfort compare with the way you felt before you saw the doctor today?
>
> 1. Much better
> 2. Somewhat better
> 3. No change
> 4. Somewhat worse
> 5. Much worse

A similar question was asked 4 or 5 days after treatment. At both time periods patients were divided into two groups: improved (1 or 2) and unimproved (3, 4, or 5).

Table VIII-1 shows the Mini-Mult standard scores of the improved and unimproved groups when the patient's immediate subjective impression was used as the measure of improvement. There were no significant differences between patients who reported immediate improvement and those who reported that their pain was unchanged or worse.

Table VIII-2 shows Mini-Mult standard scores of improved and unimproved groups when the patient's subjective impression 4 or 5 days after treatment was used as the measure of improvement. Figure VIII-1 shows the hysteria, hypochondriasis and low-back scales as predictors of both short- and long-term improvement following manipulation. In agreement with previous studies, unimproved patients showed elevated scores on Hysteria, Hypochondriasis, Psychosthenia and the low back scale. It should be noted that, as compared to the data shown in Table VIII-1, (a) the patient population is smaller because some patients did not return to the clinic and (b) the proportion of patients reporting improvement is substantially less. The latter finding is consistent with previous reports that manipulation may often produce immediate relief followed by a gradual return of the painful condition over a period of days (Fisk, 1977). This return of pain appears to be more likely in patients with "neurotic" Mini-Mult profiles.

Table VIII-1

MINI-MULT STANDARD SCORES AS A FUNCTION OF IMPROVEMENT IMMEDIATELY FOLLOWING MANIPULATION (MEANS ± STANDARD DEVIATION)

	Improved (N = 75) Mean (SD)	Not Improved (N = 14) Mean (SD)	*t*
Lie (L)	53 (8)	55 (7)	.60
Unusual Items (F)	56 (8)	53 (6)	1.17
Defensiveness (K)	54 (9)	57 (9)	1.34
Hypochondriasis (Hs)	63 (11)	63 (10)	.16
Depression (D)	65 (14)	67 (8)	.61
Hysteria (Hy)	67 (8)	68 (8)	.19
Psychopathic Deviate (Pd)	67 (11)	71 (7)	1.48
Paranoia (Pa)	60 (9)	58 (6)	.64
Psychasthenia (Pt)	59 (12)	61 (9)	.50
Schizophrenia (Sc)	64 (11)	63 (9)	.48
Mania (Ma)	57 (9)	56 (6)	1.19
Low Back Pain (Lb)	58 (11)	60 (10)	.36

From Hoehler and Tobis (1983)

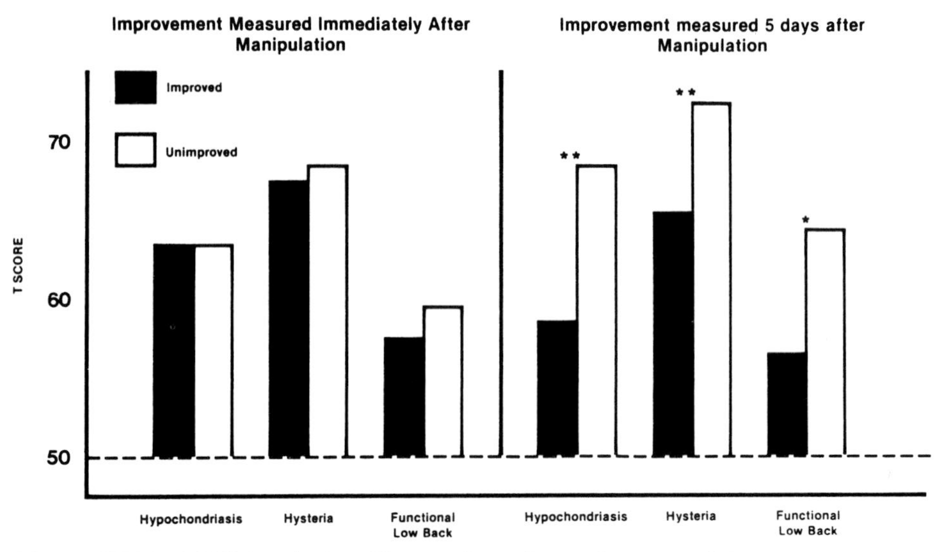

Figure VIII-1. MMPI-equivalent T scores in patients who reported improvement vs. patients who reported no improvement from manipulative therapy (from Tobis and Hoehler, 1983).

Age and sex were uncorrelated with the response to spinal manipulation at either interval. Prior duration of back pain was not correlated with immediate relief but patients reporting longer-term relief tended to have lower pain durations than those patients who did not obtain relief.

Table VIII-3 shows MMPI scores and pain durations when patient groups are subdivided according to both immediate and long-term improvement. Despite the small number of patients who were never improved or who showed delayed improvement, it is apparent that there was no interaction between short-term and long-term improvement. That is, patients who were never improved were no different from patients who displayed initial improvement followed by a relapse.

These data indicate that patients who fail to show relatively long-lasting improvement from a single spinal manipulation tend to have elevated scores on several measures of neuroticism and anxiety as well as elevated scores on the functional low back scale. However, the psychological factors measured here displayed no association with the immediate pain relief produced by manipulative therapy.

These data tend to support the "pain-fear" hypothesis proposed by Caldwell and Chase (1977). Manipulation may produce immediate relief from back pain by relieving muscle tension and restoring mobility but, in the neurotic and anxious patient, the pathological immobility may return. These patients may require a series of treatments to break the

Table VIII-2

MINI-MULT STANDARD SCORES AS A FUNCTION OF IMPROVEMENT APPROXIMATELY FIVE DAYS AFTER MANIPULATION (MEANS ± STANDARD DEVIATIONS)

Number of patient	Improved (N = 34) Mean (SD)	Not Improved (N = 28) Mean (SD)	*t*
Lie (L)	53 (8)	53 (8)	.19
Unusual Items (F)	56 (7)	56 (7)	.44
Defensiveness (K)	53 (9)	56 (7)	1.30
Hypochondriasis (Hs)	59 (10)	68 (10)	3.29 **
Depression (D)	66 (14)	68 (12)	.61
Hysteria (Hy)	65 (7)	72 (8)	3.11 **
Psychopathic Deviate (Pd)	66 (12)	71 (10)	1.67
Paranoia (Pa)	58 (10)	60 (9)	.79
Psychasthenia (Pt)	57 (13)	64 (12)	2.08 *
Schizophrenia (Sc)	63 (11)	67 (10)	1.60
Mania (Ma)	58 (10)	58 (8)	.09
Low Back Pain (Lb)	56 (12)	64 (11)	2.82 **

* $p < .05$
** $p < .01$

From Hoehler and Tobis (1983)

cycle characterized by "pain-fear" leading to immobility resulting in increased pain and fear. However, one should also consider the possibility that elevated scores on neuroticism and anxiety scales may represent a response to back pain rather than its cause. Thus, one could hypothesize that patients with nonpsychogenic back pain might, after repeated evidence that medical treatment cannot relieve their pain, develop elevated levels of anxiety and concern for bodily processes. Brena, et al (1980) have reported some tendency for MMPI score elevations to decline following successful treatment and Beals and Hickman (1972) have reported increases in Hs and Hy and decreases in D as an acute back pain becomes chronic.

Table VIII-3

MINI-MULT STANDARD SCORES AND PAIN DURATIONS (LOG_{10}) AS A FUNCTION OF BOTH IMMEDIATE AND LONG-TERM IMPROVEMENT

	Improved[1] (N = 32) Mean (SD)	Delayed Improvement[2] (N = 2) Mean (SD)	Relapsed[3] (N = 21) Mean (SD)	No Improvement[4] (N = 6) Mean (SD)
Hs	60 (10)	51 (4)	68 (11)	66 (8)
Hy	66 (8)	60 (2)	72 (9)	70 (8)
Pt	57 (13)	57 (13)	64 (13)	63 (12)
Lb	56 (12)	49 (6)	64 (10)	62 (10)
Duration	1.4 (0.6)	1.3 (0.4)	1.8 (0.7)	1.7 (0.8)

[1] Both immediate and long-term improvement

[2] Long-term improvement only

[3] Short-term improvement only

[4] No improvement at any time interval

From Hoehler and Tobis (1983)

It appears that psychological factors are an important consideration predicting the efficacy of spinal manipulation for low back pain. Patients characterized as "neurotic" may tend to show a transient improvement followed by a relapse several days after treatment.

Conclusion

Based upon the material that has been presented in previous chapters, the data should help the physician in determining which patient is likely to be benefited by manipulation therapy.

It would appear that patients with pain of relatively recent origin—in contrast to chronic duration—are relatively more responsive to manipulation.

Further, based on the study of Nwuga (1982), patients whose straight leg raising tests show marked restrictions seem to respond more dramatically than those with minimal losses in range.

For these patients who appear to be emotionally more stable, the long-term effects of manipulation would more likely be salutory.

Finally, based upon our own studies, these patients who are examined by an experienced manipulator and found to be good candidates for manipulation, will likely have a more successful outcome.

On the other hand, there is extensive evidence in the literature suggesting that many parameters are of no discriminating difference in determining efficacy of manipulation. These include: age, sex, location of pain, and abrupt or gradual onset.

CHAPTER IX

THE FUTURE

WHAT IS THE FUTURE for manipulation as a therapeutic modality? What directions shall research take relative to future studies that may be undertaken?

One can with confidence predict that manipulation will continue to be employed in the vast array of musculoskeletal complaints for which it has been used for centuries. The fact that there is a large and ever growing army of clinicians who believe themselves qualified to treat these aches and pains of mankind by this modality will insure its continued use. But, more than that, patients often find relief of discomfort by the laying-on-of-hands. In addition, the risk of complications or harmful effects is small indeed. In light of the fact that medical care is costly, that physicians are generally very busy with relatively less time available per patient than other groups of health care providers and that the use of pharmaceutical agents is potentially more toxic with greater risk of complications than manual therapy, it is likely that manipulation will grow in popularity in America in the remainder of this century.

The factors that may militate against this development are (1) if the health care system enables physicians to spend more time with patients, (2) if new drugs or nonmanipulative procedures are found to be more effective in the relief of back pain, (3) if research establishes unequivocally that manipulation is without therapeutic benefit. None of these events is likely to occur. Certainly, in regard to research, most studies to date tend to suggest that there is a measurable therapeutic effect from manipulative intervention.

What are some of the directions along which research in this field may proceed?

1) Clinical studies which are controlled and single blind have begun to appear and more are likely in the years ahead. Hopefully, these may

provide not only confirmation of the efficacy of manipulation, but also, more selectively, the types of backache for which this modality is most effective.

2) Epidemiological studies need to be developed not only in terms of incidence and prevalence of low back pain but describing the characteristics of those complaints relative to duration, age, sex and site.
3) Neurophysiological studies must be conducted employing some of the advanced technologies of science in understanding the mechanisms for low back pain. These might include (a) Thermography—for determining local changes in temperature regulation over the site of pain; (b) Impedance Plethysmography—measuring local blood flow over the site of pain; (c) Electromyography techniques—including electrical potentials over the area of pain as well as the contralateral sites without pain; H reflex to determine abnormalities in the latency resulting from the local pathology; somatosensory evoked potentials to determine if there is a prolongation of such relfexes initiated by the pain; (d) Radiographic techniques such as the CAT scan, PET scan and/or Magnetic Resonance Imaging devices (e.g. Bell et al, 1984). These newer developments may help us to either identify local morphologic changes, metabolic disorders or changes in perfusion at the site of discomfort.

How many of these may prove to be useful remains for the future to disclose. How many may only obfuscate with a plethora of data which does not elucidate the mechanism of back pain nor the means by which manipulation eradicates the complaint also remains a continuing source of speculation.

REFERENCES

Adams T, Steinmetz MA, Hersey SR, Holmes KR, Greenmon PE, Physiologic basis for skin properties in palpatory physical diagnosis. *J. Am. Osteop. Assoc.*, 81:366-370, 1982.

Agarwall A, Lloyd KN, Douey P, Thermography of the spine and sacroiliac joints in spondylitis. *Rheumatol. Phys. Med.*, 10:349-355, 1970.

Albert SM, Glickman H, Kalish M, Thermography in orthopedics. *Ann. NY Acad. Sci.*, 121:157-170, 1964.

Armstrong JR, *Lumbar Disc Lesions: Pathogenesis and Treatment of Low Back Pain and Sciatica.* E & S Livingstone, London, 1952.

Arroyo P, Electromyography in the evaluation of reflex muscle spasm. *J. Fla. Med. Assoc.*, 53:29-31, 1966.

Basmajian J, Cyclobenzaprine hydrochloride effect on skeletal muscle spasm in the lumbar region and neck: two double-blind controlled clinical and laboratory studies. *Arch. Phys. Med. Rehabilitation,* 59:58-63, 1978.

Beal M, Teaching of basic principles of osteopathic manipulative techniques. *Am. Osteop. Assn.*, 81:607-609, 1982.

Beal MC, Goodridge JP, Johnston WL, McConnell DC, Interexaminer agreement in patient improvement after a negotiated selection of tests. *J. Am. Osteop. Assoc.*, 79:432-440, 1980.

Beals RK, Hickman NW, Industrial injuries of the back and extremities. Comprehensive evaluation—An aid in the prognosis and management; A study of one hundred and eighty patients. *J. Bone Joint Surg.*, 54-A:1593-1611, 1972.

Bell GR, Rothmon RH, Booth RE, Cuckler JM, Garfin S, Herkowitz H, Simeone FA, Dolinskos C, Han SS, A study of computer assisted tomography II Comparison of metrizamide myelography and computed tomography in the diagnosis of herniated lumbar disc and spinal stenosis. *Spine*, 9:552-556, 1984.

Bergquist-Ullman M, Larsson U, Acute low back pain in industry: A controlled prospective study with special reference to therapy of confounding factors. *Act. Orthop Scand.* (Suppl), 170:1-177, 1977.

Blumetti AE, Modesti LM, Psychological predictors of success or failure of surgical intervention for intractable back pain. In J Bonica and D Able-Fessard (Eds), *Advances in Pain Research and Therapy,* Vol. 2, Raven Press, New York, pp. 323-325, 1977.

Boag AG, Manipulation in treatment of low back pain. *Br. Med. J.*, 2:334, 1975.

Bobinac-Greorgievski A, Muftic O, Electromyographic activity in erector spinae muscles during body bending movements in patients with low back pain. *EEG Clin Neurophysiol.*, 52:S146, 1981.

Bordley J, Harvey A, *Two Centuries of American Medicine.* W.B. Saunders Co., Philadelphia, 1976.

Braddom RI, Johnson CW, Standardization of H reflex and diagnostic use in S_1 radiculopathy. *Arch. Phys. Med. Rehab.*, 55:161-166, 1974.

Brena S, Wolf S, Chapman S, and Hammonds S, Chronic back pain: electromyographic, motion and behavioral assessments following sympathetic nerve block and placebos. *Pain* 8:1-10, 1980.

Buerger AA, A controlled trial of rotational manipulation in low back pain. *Manuelle Medicine,* 2:17-26, 1980.

Buerger AA, Experimental neuromuscular models of spinal manual techniques. *Manual Medicine,* 1:10-17, 1983.

Buerger AA, Tobis JS, *Approaches to the Validation of Manipulation Therapy,* Charles C Thomas. Springfield, IL, 1977.

Cailliet R, *Low Back Pain Syndrome,* 2nd ed., Davis Co., Philadelphia, 1968.

Caldwell AB, Chase C, Diagnosis and treatment of personality factors in chronic low back pain. *Clin. Orth. Rel. Res.*, 129:141-149, 1977.

Chrisman OD, Mittnach T, Snook GA, A study of the results following rotary manipulation in the lumbar intervertebral-disc syndrome. *J. Bone Joint Surg.*, 46A:517-524, 1964.

Cloward RB, The clinical significance of the sinuvertebral nerve of the cervical spine in relation to the cervical disk syndrome. *J. Neural. Neurosurg. Psychiat.*, 23:321-324, 1960.

Cobb CR, De Vries HA, Urban RT, et al., Electrical Activity in muscle pain. *Am. J. Phys. Med.*, 51:80-87, 1975.

Collins GA, Cohen MJ, Naliboff BD, Schandler SC, Comparative analysis of paraspinal and frontalis EMG, heart rate and skin conductance in chronic low back pain. *J. Rehab. Med.*, 14:39-46, 1982.

Coxhead CE, Inskip H, Meade TW, North WRS, Troup JDG, Multicentre trial of physiotherapy in the management of sciatic symptoms. *Lancet,* 1:1065-1068, 1981.

Coyer AB, Curwen IHM, Low back pain treated by manipulation: A controlled series. *Brit. Med. J.*, 1:705-707, 1955.

Crelin BS, A scientific test of the chiropractic theory. *American Scientist,* 61:574-580, 1973.

Crown S, Psychological aspects of low back pain. *Rheum. Rehab.*, 17:114-124, 1978.

Cyriax J, *Textbook of Orthopedic Medicine Vol. I.* Baillier Tindall, London, 1982.

Cyriax J, *Textbook of Orthopedic Medicine Vol. II.* Williams & Wilkins, Baltimore, 1971.

Cyriax JH, Manipulation in treatment of low back pain. *Br. Med. J.*, 2:334, 1975.

Denslow JS, Hassett CC, The central excitatory state associated with postural abnormalities. *J. Neurophysiol.*, 5:393-402, 1942.

Denslow JS, Pathophysiologic Evidence for the Osteopathic Lesion. Data on what is known, what is not known, and what is controversial. In. M. Goldstein (Ed.), *The Research Status of Spinal Manipulative Therapy,* DHEW Publication No. (NIH) 76-998. Bethesda, MD, pp 227-234, 1975.

Deschuytere J, Rosselle N, Electromyographic and neurophysiological investigation in root compression syndromes in man. *Electromyography,* 10:339-340, 1970.
De Vries HA, Electromyographic observation of the effect of static stretching upon muscular distress. *Res. Quart.,* 32:468-479, 1961.
De Vries HA, Quantitiative electromyographic investigation of the spasm theory of muscular pain. *Amer. J. Phys. Med.,* 45:119-134, 1966.
De Vries HA, EMG fatigue curves in postural muscles. A possible etiology for ideopathic low back pain. *Am. J. Phys. Med.,* 47:175-181, 1968.
Deyo RA, Conservative therapy in low back pain: Distinguishing useful from useless therapy. *JAMA,* 250:1057-1-62, 1983.
Dixon A, Diagnosis of low back pain—sorting the complainers. In Jayson M (ed) *The Lumbar Spine and Back Pain.* Grune & Stratton, New York, 1976.
Doran DML, Newell DJ, Manipulation in the treatment of low back pain: A multicentre study. *Br. Med. J.,* 2:161-164, 1975.
Dvorak J, Manual medicine in the United States and Europe in the year 1982. *Manual Medicine,* 1:3-9, 1983.
Ebbetts J, Manipulation in treatment of low back pain. *Br. Med. J.,* 2:393, 1975.
Edeikin J, Wallace JD, Curley RF, et al, Thermography and herniated lumbar disks. *Am J. Roentgen.,* 102:790-796, 1968.
Edwards BC, Low back pain and pain resulting from lumbar spine conditions: A comparison of treatment results. *Austrl. J. Physiotherapy,* 15:104-110, 1969.
Elliot RA, Tender muscles in sciatica. *Lancet,* 1:47-49, 1944.
Evans DP, Burke MS, Lloyd KN, et al, Lumbar spinal manipulation on trial, Part I—clinical assessment. *Rheumatol. Rehabil.,* 17:46-53, 1978.
Fahrni WH, Observations on straight leg raising with special reference to nerve root adhesions. *Canadian J. Sur.,* 9:44-48, 1966.
Falconer MA, McGeorge M, Begg ACG: Observations on the cause and mechanism of symptom production in sciatica and low back pain. *J. Neurol. Neurosurg. Psychiat,* 11:13-26, 1948.
Farrell J, Twomey L, Acute low back pain: comparison of two conservative treatment approaches. *Med. J. Aust.,* 1:160-164, 1982.
Finneson BE, Modulating effect of secondary gain on the low back pain syndrome. In J Bonica and D Albe-Fessard (Eds), *Advances in Pain Research and Therapy, Vol. l,* Raven Press, New York, pp 949-952, 1976.
Firman G, Goldstein M, The Furtue of Chiropractic: A Psychosocial View. *N. Eng J. Med.,* 293:639-642, 1975.
Fisher MA, Shivde AJ, Teixera C, Grainen LS, Clinical and electrophysiological appraisal of the significance of radicular injury in back pain. *J. Neurol. Neurosurg. Psychiat.,* 41:303-306, 1978.
Fisk JW, Manipulation in general practice. *N.E. Med. J.,* 74:172-175, 1971.
Fisk JW, The straight-leg raising test—its relevance to possible disc pathology. *N. Z. Med. J.,* 81:557-560, 1975.
Fisk JW, An evaluation of manipulation in the treatment of the acute low back pain syndrome in general practice in A Buerger and J Tobis (eds) *Approaches to the Validation of Manipulation Therapy.* Charles C Thomas, Springfield, IL, pp 236-270, 1977, (a).
Fisk JW, *The Painful Neck and Back.* Charles C Thomas, Springfield, IL, 1977, (b).

Fisk JW, The passive hamstring stretch test: A comparison of clinical estimates with tension gauge measurements. *N.Z. Med. J.*, 89:346-348, 1979, (a).

Fisk JW, A controlled trial of manipulation in a selected group of patients with low back pain favoring one side. *N. Z. J. Med.*, 90:288-291, 1979, (b).

Flor H, Turk DC, Etiological theories and treatments for chronic back pain I. Somatic Models and interventions. *Pain*, 19:105-121, 1984.

Ford LT, Clinical use of chymopapain in lumbar and dorsal disk lesions. An end-result study. *Clin. Orthop.*, 67:81-87, 1969.

Frymoyer J, Hanley E, Howe J, et al, Disc Excision and Spine Fusion in the Management of Lumbar Disc Disease. *Spine* 3:1-6, 1978.

Frymoyer J, Matteri R, Hanley E, Failed Lumbar Disc Surgery Requiring Second Operation: A Long Term Follow-Up Study. *Spine* 3:7-11, 1978.

Glover JR, Morris JG, Khosla T, Back pain: A randomized clinical trial of rotational manipulation of the trunk. *Br. J. Ind. Med.*, 31:59-64, 1974.

Glover JR, Back pain and hyperaesthesia. Loncet, 1:1165-1169, 1960.

Godfrey CM, Morgan PP, Schatzken J, A randomized trial of manipulation for low back pain in a medical setting. *Spine*, 9:301-304, 1984.

Goldberg HI, Heinz ER, Taveras J, Thermography in the neurologic patient. *Acta Radiol*, 5:786f-795, 1966.

Goldstein M, Introduction, Summary, and Analysis in M Goldstein (Ed.) *The Research Status of Spinal Manipulative Therapy*, DHEW. Publication No. (NIH) 76-998, Bethesda, MD, 1975.

Goldthwait JE, Lumbosacral Articulation. *Boston Med. Surg. Journal*, 164:365, 1911.

Gowers W, Lumbago: Its Lesions and Analogues. Brit. Med. Jour., 1:117-121, 1904.

Greenland S, Reisbord LS, Haldeman DC, Buerger AA, Controlled clinical trials of manipulation: A review and a proposal. *J. Occup. Med.*, 22:670-676, 1980.

Grieve G, Manipulation Therapy for Neck Pain. *Physiotherapy*, 65:136-146, 1979.

Gunby P, Study to evaluate manipulation therapy. *JAMA*, 249:3148-3150, 1983.

Gunn CC, Chir B, Milbrandt WE, Tenderness at motor points. A diagnostic and prognostic aid for low-back injury. *J. Bone Jt. Surg.*, 58A:815-825, 1976.

Gunn CC, Chir B, Milbrandt E, Early and subtle signs in low back sprain. *Spine*, 3:267-281, 1978.

Haldeman S, Chiropractic Needs Proper Diagnosis. *Canadian Med. Assn. J.*, 116:593, 1977, (a).

Haldeman S, What Is Meant By Manipulation?, in A Buerger and J Tobis, (Eds.), *Approaches to the Validation of Manipulation Therapy*, Charles C Thomas, Springfield, IL, pp 299-302, 1977.

Haldeman S, Spinal manipulative therapy in the management of low back pain. In Finneson B, (Ed.) *Low Back Pain*, J. B. Lippincott Co., Philadelphia, pp 245-275, 1980.

Hanvik LJ, MMPI profiles in patients with low back pain. *J. Consult. Clin. Psychol.*, 15:350-353, 1951.

Hirsch C, Etiology and pathogenesis of low back pain. *Isr. J. Med. Sci.*, 2:362-270, 1966.

Hirsch C, An attempt to diagnose the level of a disc lesion clinically by disc puncture. *Acta Ortho Scand*, 18:132, 1978.

Hoag, JM, Basic Considerations, In Hoag, JM, Cole, WV, and Bradford, SG (Eds.), *Osteopathic Medicine,* McGraw Hill, New York, 1969.

Hoehler FK, Facilitation of the H-reflex in low back pain. *Electromyogr. Clin. Neurophysiol.,* 21:207-212, 1981.

Hoehler FK, Tobis JS, Buerger AA, Spinal Manipulation for low back pain, *JAMA,* 245:1835-1838, 1981.

Hoehler FK, Tobis JS, Low back pain and its treatment by spinal manipulation: Measures or flexibility and asymmetry. *Rheumatol. Rehabil.,* 21:21-26, 1982.

Hoehler FK, Tobis JS, Psychological factors in the treatment of back pain by spinal manipulation. *Br. J. Rheumatol.,* 22:206-212, 1983.

Holt EP, The question of lumbar discography. *J. Bone Jt. Surg,* 50:720-726, 1968.

Horal J, The Clinical appearance of low back disorders in the City of Gothenberg, Sweden. *Acta Arth. Scan.,* Suppl. No. 118, pp 68-79, 1969.

Hoyt WH, Hunt H, De Pauw M, et al, Electromyographic assessment of chronic low back pain syndrome. *J. Am. Osteo. Assn.,* 80:728-730, 1981.

Hult L, Cervical Dorsal and Lumbar Spinal Syndromes. *Acta Orthopaedica Scandinavica,* Suppl. 17, pp 96-102, 1954.

Javid MJ, Nordby EJ, Ford LJ, Heyna WJ, et al, Safety and efficacy of Chymopapain (Chymodiactin) in herniated nucleus pulposus with sciatica. *JAMA,* 249, 2489-2494, 1983.

Jayasinghe M, Harding R, Anderson J and Sweetman B, An electromyographic investigation of postural fatigue in low back pain—a preliminary study. *Electromyogr. Clin. Neurophysiol.,* 18:191-198, 1978.

Jayson M, Sims-Williams H, Young S, et al, Mobilization and manipulation for low back pain. *Spine* 6:409-416, 1981.

Johnston WL, Beal MC, Blum GA et al, Passive gross motion testing: Part III. Examiner agreement on selected subjects. *J. Am. Osteop. Assoc.,* 81:309-313, 1982.

Johnston WL, Elkiss ML, Marino RV, Blum GA, Passive gross motion testing: Part II. A study of interexaminer agreement. *J. Am. Osteop. Assoc.,* 81:304-308, 1982.

Johnston WL, Hill JL, Elkiss ML, Marino RV, A statistical model for evaluating stability of palpatory cues. *J. Am. Osteop. Assoc.,* 77:473-474, 1978.

Kamihira M, The evoked electromyographic stuidies of low back pain, especially in connection with the nerve conduction velocity of the tibial nerve. *Electromyography,* 8:191-193, 1968.

Kane RL, Leymaster C, Olsen D, Woolley FR, Fisher ED, Manipulating the patient: A comparison of the effectiveness of physician and chiropractor care. *Lancet,* 2:1333-1336, 1974.

Keim H, Kikaldy-Willis WH, Low-back pain. *Clinical Symposia vol. 32,* 1980.

Kellgren JH, Observations on referred pain arising from muscle. *Clinical Science,* 3:175-190, 1939.

Kewalramani L, Orth M, Kewalramani D, Krebs M, and Saleem A, Myelopathy following cervical spine manipulation. *Am. J. Phys. Med.,* 61:165-175, 1982.

Kincannon JC, Prediction of the standard MMPI scale scores from 71 items: The Mini-Mult. *J. Consult. Clin. Psychol.,* 32:319-335, 1968.

Kirkaldy-Willis WH, Manipulation, in Kirkaldy-Willis WH (Ed.), *Managing Low Back Pain,* Churchill Livingstone, New York, pp 175-183, 1983.

Korr IM, *The Neurobiologic Mechanims in Manipulative Therapy.* Plenum Press, New York, 1978.

Korr IM, Wright HM, Chuce JA, Cutaneous patterns of sympathetic activity in clinical abnormalities of the musculoskeletal system. *Acta Neurovegetativa,* 25:589-606, 1964.

Korr IM, Wright HM, Thomas PE, Effect of Experimental myofacial insults on cutaneous patterns of sympathetic activity in man. *Acta Neurovegetativa,* 23:329-355, 1962.

Kraft GH, Johnson EW, La Bon MM, The fibrositis syndrome. *Arch. Phys. Med.,* 49:155-162, 1968.

Kravitz E, Moore ME, Glaros A, Paralumbar muscle activity in chronic low back pain. *Arch. Phys. Med. Rehab.,* 62:172-176, 1981.

Krueger B, and Okazaki H, Vertebral-basilar distribution infarction following chiropractic cervical manipulation. *Mayo Clinic Proceedings,* 55:322-332, 1980.

Lankhorst CJ, van de Stadt RJ, Vogelaar TW, van der Korst JK, Prevo AJH, Objectivity and repeatability of measurements in low back pain.

Lewit K, The contribution of clinical observation to neurobiological mechanisms in manipulation therapy. in Korr IM, ed., *The Neurobiologic Mechanisms in Manipulative Therapy,* Plenum Press, New York, pp 3-25, 1978.

Lloyd GG, Wolkind SN, Greenwood R, Harris DJ, A psychiatric study of patients with persistent low back pain. *Rheum. Rehab.,* 18:30-34, 1979.

Loebl WY, Measurements of spinal posture and range of spinal movements. *Ann. Phys. Med.,* 9:103, 1967.

Lomax E, Manipulative therapy: An historical perspective in A Buerger and J Tobis, (Eds.) *Approaches to the Validation of Manipulative Therapy,* Charles C Thomas, Springfield, IL, pp 205-216, 1977.

Macrae I, and Wright V, Measurement of Back Movement. *Ann. Rheum. Dis,* 28:584-589, 1969.

Maigne R, *Orthopedic Medicine.* Charles C Thomas, Springfield, IL, 1972.

Maitland G, *Vertebral Manipulation.* Butterworths, London, 4th ed., 1977.

Malcolm D, A method of measuring reflex times applied in sciatica and other conditions due to nerve-root compression. *J. Neurol. Neurosurg. Psychiat.,* 14:15-24, 1951.

Matthews J, and Yates D, Reduction of Lumbar Disc Prolapse by Manipulation. Br. Med. J., 3:696-697, 1969.

McCreary C, Turner J, Dawson E, The MMPI as a predictor of response to conservative treatment for low back pain. *J. Clin. Psychol.,* 35:278-284, 1979.

McGlynn GH, Laughlin NT, Rowe BS, Effect of elecytromyographic feedback and static stretching on artificially induced muscle soreness. *Am. J. Phys. Med.,* 58:139-148, 1979.

McNab I, McCullock JA, Weiner DS, et al, Chemonucleolysis. *Can. J. Surg.,* 14:280-289, 1971.

Meyer TG, Tenier AF, Kristoferson S, Mooney V, Use of noninvasive techniques for quantification of spinal range of motion in normal subjects and chronic low-back dysfunction patients. *Spine,* 9:588-595, 1984.

Mixter WJ, and Barr JS, Ruptures of the intervertebral disc with involvement of the spinal canal. N. Eng. J. Med., 211:210, 1934.

Moran PS, Pruzzo NA, Mitchell FL, *An Evaluation and Treatment Manual of Osteopathic*

Manipulative Procedure. Institute for Continuing Education in Osteopathic Principles, Kansas City, MO, 1973.

Nachemson, AL, The lumbar spine. An orthopaedic challenge. *Spine,* 1:59-71, 1976.

Nachemson A, Evens JH, Some mechanical properties of the third human lumbar interlaminar ligament (ligamentum flavum). J. Biomech, 1:211-220, 1968.

Newell DJ, Manipulation in the treatment of low back pain: A multicenter study. in, A Buerger and J Tobis (eds). *Approaches to the Validation of Manipulation Therapy,* Charles C Thomas, Springfield, IL, pp 284-298, 1977.

Nouwen A, Bush C, The relationship between paraspinal EMG and chronic low back pain. *Pain,* 20:109-123, 1984.

Nwuga V, Relative Therapeutic Efficacy of Vertebral Manipulation and Conventional Treatment in Back Pain Management. *Am. J. Phys. Med.,* 61:6:273-278, 1982.

Nwuga VC, *Manipulation of the Spine.* Williams & Wilkins, Baltimore, 1976.

Pace J and Nagle. Piriform syndrome. *Western J. Med.,* 124:435-439, 1976.

Palmer BJ, *The Subluxation Specific—The Adjustment Specific.* Vol. 18, Palmer School of Chiropractic, Davenport, 1934.

Parker G, Prior D, Tupling H, New Zealand inquiry into chiropractic. *Med. J. Aust.,* 1:103-105, 1980.

Parker GB, Tupling H, Pryor DS, A controlled trial of cervical manipulation for migraine. *Aust. N.Z. Med.,* 8:589-593, 1978.

Peto R, Pike MC, Armitage P, Breslow NE, Cox DR, Howard SV, Mantel N, McPherson K, Peto J, Smith PG, Design and analysis of randomized clinical trials requiring prolonged observation of each patient. *Br. J. Cancer,* 34:585-612, 1976.

Pochaczevsky R, Assessment of back pain by contact thermography of extremity dermatomes. *Orthop. Rev.,* 12:45-58, 1983.

Rasmussen TG, Manipulation in treatment of low back pain (A randomized clinical trial). *Manuelle Med.,* 1:8-10, 1978.

Retzloff EW, Berry AH, Haight AS, et al, The piriformis muscle syndrome. *J. Am. Osteopath. Assoc.,* 73:799-807, 1974.

Reynolds PMG, Measurement of spinal mobility: A comparison of three methods. *Rheum. Rehabil.,* 14:180-185, 1975.

Riches E, Manipulation in treatment of back pain. *Br. Med. J.,* 2:334, 1975.

Roberts GM, Roberts EE, Lloyd KN, Lumbar spinal manipulation on trial, Part II. Radiological assessment. *Rheum. Rehabil.,* 17:54-59, 1978.

Rubal BJ, Traycoff RB, Ewing KL, Liquid Crystal Thermography. A new tool for evaluating low back pain. *Physical Therapy,* 62:1593-1596, 1982.

Sarno JE, Etiology of back and neck pain—an autonomic myoneuralgia. *J. Nerv. Ment. Dis.,* 169:55-59, 1981.

Schiotz E, and Cyriax J, *Manipulation Past and Present.* William Heinemann Medical Books Ltd., London, 1975.

Schober P, "Len denwirbelsaule under Kreuschmergen" (The Lumbar Vertebral Column and Backache). *Munch. Med. Wschr.,* 84:336, 1937.

Schuchmann JH, Reflex latency in radiculpathy. *Arch. Phys. Med. Rehabil.,* 59:185-187, 1978.

Schwetschenau PR, Ramirez A, Johnston J, et al, Double blind evaluation of intradiscal chymopapain for herniated lumbar discs. Early results. *J. Neurosurg.*, 45:622-627, 1976.

Sherman D, Hart R, and Easton J, Abrupt change in head position and cerebral infarction. *Stroke,* 12:2-6, 1981.

Silk AD, Chiropractic: A medical fortune cookie. *Bull. Orange County Med. Assn.*, 51:11, 1982.

Sims-Williams H, Jayson MIV, Young SMS, et al, Controlled clinical trial of mobilisation and manipulation for patients with low back pain in general practice. *Br. Med. J.*, 2:1338-1340, 1978.

Sims-Williams H, Jayson MIV, Young SMS, Buddeley H, Collins E, Controlled trial of mobilisation and manipulation for low back pain: hospital patients. *Br. Med. J.*, 2:1318-1320, 1979.

Sinclair D, Weddell G, Feindel W, et al, referred pain and associated phenomena. *Brain,* 71, 184, 1948.

Sloop PR, Smith DS, Goldenberg E, Dore C, Manipulation for chronic neck pain: A double-blind controlled study. *Spine* 7:532-535, 1982.

Smyth MJ, and Wright V, Sciatica and the intervertebral disc. An experimental study. *J. Bone Joint Surg.*, 40:1401-1418, 1958.

Soderberg GL, Barr JO, Muscular function in chronic low-back disfunction. *Spine,* 8:79-85, 1983.

Spangfort E, The Lumbar Disc Herniation. *Acta Orth. Scand. Supplement* No. 142, 1972.

Steindler A, The interpretation of sciatic radiation and the syndrom of low back pain. J. Bone Jt. Surg., 22:28-34, 1948.

Still AT, *Osteopathy: Research and Practice.* Kirksville, MO, 1910.

Stoddard A. *A Manual of Osteopathic Practice.* New York, Harper & Row, 1969.

Sweetman BJ, Anderson JAD, Dalton ER, The relationships between little-finger mobility, straight-leg raising and low-back pain. *Rheumatol. Rehabil.*, 13:161-166, 1974.

Swezey RL, Silverman TR, Radiographic demonstration of induced vertebral facet displacement. *Arch. Phys. Med. Rehab.*, 52:244-249, 1971.

Tichauer ER, The objective corroboration of back pain through thermography. *J. Occup. Med.*, 19:727-731, 1977.

Tobis JS, Hoehler FK, Musculoskeletal manipulation in the treatment of low back pain. *Bull. N. Y. Acad. Med.*, 59:660-668, 1983.

Travell J, and Rinzler S, The Myofascial Genesis of Pain. *Postgraduate Med.* 11:425-434, 1952.

Tsushima WT, Relationship between the Mini-Mutl and the MMPI with medical patients. *J. Clin. Psychol.*, 31:673-675, 1975.

Turk DC, Flor H, Etiological theories and treatments for chronic back pain. II. Psychological models and interventions. *Pain,* 19:209-233, 1984.

Wardwell N, *Limited, Marginal and Quasi-Practitioners. Handbook of Medical Sociology,* 2nd ed., Prentice-Hall, Inc., pp 250-273, 1972.

Ware, AC, Wilkinson JA, Burn JMB, Langdon L, Chronic lumbosciatic syndrome treated by epidural injection and manipulation. *Practitioner,* 209:53-59, 1972.

Weber H, Lumbar disc herniation: a controlled prospective study with ten years of observation. *Spine,* 8:131-140, 1983.

Wilfing FJ, Klonoff H, Kokan P, Psychological, demographic and orthopaedic factors associated with prediction of out come of spianl fusion. *Clin. Orthop. Rel. Res.*, 90:153-160, 1973.

Wilson JN, Ilfeld FW, Manipulation of the herniated intervertebral disc. *Am. J. Surg.*, 83:173, 1952.

Wiltse, LL, Rocchio PD, Preoperative psychological tests as predictors of success of chemonucleolysis in the treatment of the low back pain syndrome. *J. Bone Joint Surg.*, 57-A:478-483, 1975.

Wolkind SN, Forrest AJ, Low back pain: A psychiatric investigation. *Postgrad. Med. J.*, 48:76-79, 1972.

AUTHOR INDEX

SUBJECT INDEX

T

V